~ The ~
# PREGNANT
# GODDESS

Your Guide to
Traditions, Rituals, and Blessings
for a Sacred Pagan Pregnancy

Arin Murphy-Hiscock
Author of *The Green Witch*

ADAMS MEDIA
New York ✦ London ✦ Toronto ✦ Sydney ✦ New Delhi

Aadamsmedia

Adams Media
An Imprint of Simon & Schuster, Inc.
100 Technology Center Drive
Stoughton, Massachusetts 02072

First Adams Media hardcover edition
June 2020

ADAMS MEDIA and colophon are trademarks of Simon & Schuster.

For information about special discounts for bulk purchases, please contact Simon & Schuster Special Sales at 1-866-506-1949 or business@simonandschuster.com.

The Simon & Schuster Speakers Bureau can bring authors to your live event. For more information or to book an event contact the Simon & Schuster Speakers Bureau at 1-866-248-3049 or visit our website at www.simonspeakers.com.

Interior design and illustrations by Priscilla Yuen

Manufactured in China

10 9 8 7 6 5 4 3

Library of Congress Cataloging-in-Publication Data
Names: Murphy-Hiscock, Arin, author.
Title: The pregnant goddess / Arin Murphy-Hiscock, author of The Green Witch.
Description: Avon, Massachusetts: Adams Media, 2020. | Includes bibliographical references and index.
Identifiers: LCCN 2020002003 | ISBN 9781507213834 (hc) | ISBN 9781507213841 (ebook)
Subjects: LCSH: Pregnant women--Religious life. | Pregnancy--Religious aspects. | Mother goddesses. | Neopaganism--Customs and practices
Classification: LCC BV4529.18 .M87 2020 | DDC 299/.94--dc23
LC record available at https://lccn.loc .gov/2020002003

ISBN 978-1-5072-1383-4
ISBN 978-1-5072-1384-1 (ebook)

Contains material adapted from the following title published by Adams Media, an Imprint of Simon & Schuster, Inc.: *Pagan Pregnancy* by Arin Murphy-Hiscock, copyright © 2008, ISBN 978-1-59869-397-3.

Dedication

This one's for Pasley, Jeff, and Devon, who were there for us throughout my pregnancy and who continue to support us throughout the joys of parenthood, and for Tallis, who helped her mother review the book.

Acknowledgments

I say it every time, but it's worth repeating: No one ever writes a book in a vacuum, and my support system has, as usual, been invaluable to me. Janice and Ceri in particular were strong and encouraging throughout the writing of the first iteration of this book in 2006 and 2007, and it's the better for their efforts.

Specific thanks go out to Pasley and Colleen, who read the book in manuscript form while they were pregnant and gave me supportive feedback. It was an unlooked-for honor to be able to share the work with them when they needed it, and to share parts of it with Andrea L. as well. I'm grateful to Scarlet for always keeping her library available to me and for obtaining the Dundes book for me not once but twice! Thanks also go to Anne-Pandora, Kristin, and Andrea L. for responding to a query about their experiences, and for assuring me that I was on the right track.

My editor Andrea went to bat for me over and over to eventually secure the release of the first edition of this book as an ebook, finally allowing it to be available to readers after a long delay.

For this new edition (and first print release!), Rebecca Tarr Thomas and Brett Palana-Shanahan have been absolutely wonderful to work with, as always.

And of course, I wouldn't have been able to write about the spiritual aspects of pregnancy without Ron and Will, who gave me the opportunity in the first place.

Contents

Introduction

When a woman is pregnant, she becomes the very essence of the Goddess: she who carries life within her, she who will rebirth new life created from old.

Apart from the many physical changes, there is a whole other dimension to pregnancy—namely, that you are transitioning from one state to another, as well as creating life. *The Pregnant Goddess* will address these aspects of pregnancy and birth from a uniquely neo-pagan perspective, using rituals and meditations to help you attune to the energies that shift throughout your pregnancy.

Inside you'll discover:

* ❖ How to handle working with energies responsibly while pregnant
* ❖ How to deal with emotional changes
* ❖ Rituals to protect your pregnancy and baby
* ❖ How to use your faith to address unexpected events
* ❖ Which herbs and oils are safe to use while pregnant and which should be avoided

- ❖ Tips for preparing your home and life for your new arrival
- ❖ How to make time for your spiritual practice after the baby is born

Of course, your medical professional will be the key person to work with to get a handle on the physical changes that are, or will soon be, occurring in your pregnancy. But your doctor can't necessarily help with the spiritual struggle you'll be working through. In the midst of such an incredible life-changing event, you'll need to turn to your gods and goddesses, your faith, and your practice to make sense of the spiritual shifts and fluctuations that pregnancy brings along with it—and this book will show you how to do just that.

In these pages you will find the comfort, relief, and guidance you will need to embrace your inner goddess; she will help you carry yourself with ease into this next exciting stage of life.

❖ ❖ ❖

Chapter 1

Preparations and Beginnings

Pregnancy can be an intimidating experience. No matter how many books you read, no matter how much anecdotal advice you hear from other women who have been pregnant, going through it yourself for the first time, or any time at all, is a big deal.

It is important to think of pregnancy as a process, not a condition. One doesn't catch pregnancy and then recover from it. Pregnancy changes you and your life on a deep level. You can never go back. It is a life-changing experience, one that seems to last forever and yet is over so quickly.

You spend so much time while pregnant worrying, making appointments, trying to balance work with your daily life and the new demands your body makes of you. But in this chapter you will learn how important it is to take the time to simply sit and experience your pregnancy and to explore the sensations, the meaning, the energy, and the gifts this process brings to you.

Spiritual Preparation for Pregnancy

Is anyone truly ready for pregnancy?

On the surface of that question is the obvious answer: If you can conceive or have conceived, then you are physiologically ready for the state of pregnancy.

Whether you are mentally, emotionally, or spiritually ready, well, that's another story. Even if you have previously been pregnant, that experience serves only as a guideline for how this pregnancy will go and how you will feel and react to the changes in your body once again. It is one of the miracles of pregnancy that every experience with it will be different. Every gestation is unique and you must look to the beginning, to the moment of fertilization, to trace the slow shifts and evolutions in your energy and your spirituality.

Spiritually preparing for pregnancy, whether you have the opportunity to do it before you conceive or when you discover that you have already done so, allows you to clear the decks, so to speak; it allows you to sweep away unnecessary baggage and obstacles in order to focus on this new state into which you are moving. It offers the opportunity to tidy up and make room in your emotional and spiritual life for this new idea, this new reality.

How you go about spiritually preparing for pregnancy will depend on you as an individual and on what point in the process you have reached. Are you already pregnant and seeking to encompass that new reality? Are you looking to become pregnant and preparing yourself mentally and spiritually for the venture?

Spiritually preparing for pregnancy can include:

❖ Attuning to your own body's physical cycle: being aware of your menstrual cycle and how your body reacts to the seasons, to the weather, and to physical environments.

❖ Attuning to your own emotional cycle: being aware of how your emotional state is impacted by the physical environment and interpersonal situations.

❖ Meditating on the spiritual implications of motherhood: What does being a mother mean to you? What is your perception of the ideal mother? What kind of relationship have you had with your mother? With other mothers of your acquaintance?

❖ Meditating on the part of your life that is drawing to an end. (Modern paganism commonly interprets the Goddess as manifesting in the triple aspect of Maiden-Mother-Crone. With your first pregnancy, you explore the physical definition of the Mother aspect. The aspects of the Goddess and what they represent will be examined in Chapter 3.)

Creating a Pregnancy Shrine

As part of your spiritual preparation for pregnancy, creating a place where you can focus your thoughts and energies outside yourself can be helpful. The point of the pregnancy shrine is to give you the opportunity to pay attention for a while to the process of your pregnancy, rather than its outcome (the baby). It will serve as a place of focus for your own changes, a place to celebrate you.

Select a suitable location to set up your shrine: your bedside table, a small wall shelf, a shelf on a bookcase, an end table—somewhere where you will see it and be able to interact with it regularly. Throughout your pregnancy the shrine will likely collect other items, so make sure it's somewhere that can accommodate that future assortment of meaningful objects.

This project includes making a collage. Before you begin, find pictures of pregnant women. Look them up on the Internet and print them out, go through pregnancy magazines, look in catalogs and flyers, and look at art and photography postcards. Choose pictures that inspire you, that make you feel happy, confident, strong, feminine, awed, or anything positive that you associate with pregnancy. Collect these pictures in a folder.

Your collage should be framed. A small picture frame, either 4" × 6" or 5" × 7", is usually more convenient to fit on your shrine. If you have a large enough shrine space, you can use an 8" × 10" frame if you like. If one is not included in the frame, prepare a sheet of cardboard or card stock to fit inside the frame upon which to make your collage.

YOU WILL NEED

- ❖ Folder of pictures of pregnant women
- ❖ Scissors
- ❖ Sheet of cardboard or card stock to fit inside the frame
- ❖ Glue
- ❖ Sealant and a brush (or a spray sealant) (optional)
- ❖ Small picture frame
- ❖ Seashell(s)
- ❖ Small cup or chalice

- ❖ Small incense burner (for sticks, cones, or charcoal—select the one that will serve you best, according to your tastes and preference)
- ❖ Small votive candle and holder
- ❖ Small dish of salt, sand, or earth (preferably earthenware or ceramic)
- ❖ Scarf, cloth, or doily (optional)

DIRECTIONS

1. Cut out the pictures and arrange them on a sheet of cardboard or card stock in a pleasing arrangement. Glue them down. If you are concerned about fading or peeling, brush or spray a layer of sealant over the collage. When it is dry, place the collage in the frame.

2. Arrange the elemental representations on your shrine in a pleasing grouping. Make sure you will be able to reach the candle without knocking anything over and that the flame of the candle and coal of the incense will not interfere with anything above or around the shrine.

3. Put the framed collage on your shrine.

4. Hold your hands over the shrine palms down, and say:

   I call upon the universe to consecrate this shrine.
   Come air, come fire, come water, come earth
   And bless this place.
   May it offer me joy and introspection,
   Calm and tranquility,
   As I pass through the transformations and growth
   Of my pregnancy.
   Mother Goddess, bless this shrine with your love for me and
   *   all living things.*
   Thank you.
   So may it be.

5. If you would like to write your own prayer for consecrating your shrine, then by all means do so. Your words will resonate with your own spirit and be more meaningful to you.

6. As you acquire other significant items during your pregnancy—perhaps the test that confirms your pregnancy, a stone you pick up, cards or letters, spell sachets and charms—place them on the shrine as well. Don't start out by gathering a bunch of items to fill the shrine or you'll rapidly run out of space; let them slowly come to you over the nine calendar months of your journey.

7. If at any time you feel something no longer has a place on your shrine and that its purpose has been fulfilled, remove it with respect. Dispose of it by burying it if it is biodegradable or by burning it and scattering the ashes outdoors; if it is not, recycle it or pass it on in some way to someone else who can use it. If it has been empowered, disempower it before you discard it by holding it in your hands and enacting the empowering process in reverse: Allow the item's energy to flow back into you, as if you were drinking it in. If you do not wish to absorb the item's energy, place it on the ground so that the earth can absorb any energy, or leave it in the sink under running water if the water won't destroy it, or place it in sunlight for a day or in moonlight for a night.

Blessing the Decision to Conceive

If you have decided to conceive a child, you have the opportunity to bless the venture before you begin.

Beeswax is preferred here for its natural origins, but it can be challenging to find noncolored beeswax candles. If you have trouble finding them, simply use the palest beeswax candle that you can find. Your candle should be small for this ritual, as beeswax burns slowly. A birthday candle, a tealight, or a 4" taper are all ideal choices.

YOU WILL NEED

- ❖ Small white beeswax taper candle (see previous note)
- ❖ Candleholder
- ❖ Matches or a lighter
- ❖ Sandalwood incense
- ❖ Incense burner
- ❖ Small cup or chalice of water
- ❖ Small dish of earth, sand, or salt
- ❖ Approximately $\frac{1}{4}$ cup (or 1 heaping tablespoon) dried lavender flowers (alternatively, sprigs of fresh lavender)
- ❖ 1 tablespoon frankincense tears
- ❖ Moonstone
- ❖ Small square of cotton or silk
- ❖ Length of pale green cotton yarn or embroidery floss

DIRECTIONS

1. Center and ground. (See Chapter 5 for a discussion of these techniques.)

2. Create sacred space as per your customary practice. If you wish, you may invoke the elements.

3. Invoke Divinity:

   Sacred Mother
   From whose womb all life comes,
   Bless me as I set out upon this path.
   Make me a vessel of life, of hope, of love.
   Grant me the serenity to embrace my fertility

And to acknowledge the Divine power that rests
  within my own womb.
Sacred Mother
I am your daughter
And your daughter welcomes your blessing.
So may it be.

4. Sit or stand at your altar and light the candle, saying:

   I light this candle as a token of my wish to be a bearer of light
     throughout the coming time.
   Element of fire, lend me your warmth.
   Illuminate me with the essence of life, the warmth of growth.
   And may your flame guide me through challenges to come.

5. Light the incense, saying:

   Element of air, I call upon you to flow through my life.
   Keep my thoughts flowing freely, my energy free.

6. Pick up the cup or chalice of water and raise it to your lips for a sip, saying:

   Element of water, I call upon you to lend me your healing
     energies.
   Help me to be in the best of health throughout the coming
     time.
   Teach me to accept my emotions and to embrace the coming
     changes.

7. Touch your fingertips to the earth, sand, or salt, saying:

   Element of earth, lend me your stability.
   Help keep me grounded through the coming time.
   Teach me to move in harmony with the fertile Earth herself.

8. Move the candle so that it sits in the center of the altar. Sprinkle the lavender around it, or if you have fresh sprigs of the herb, arrange them around the candleholder, saying:

   Lavender, I call upon your peacefulness now.
   Lend to me your purity and tranquility.

9. Take the frankincense tears in your hands and sprinkle them on the lavender, saying:

   Frankincense, I call upon your serenity now.
   Lend to me your joy and strength.

10. Take the moonstone in your hands, saying:

    Moonstone, I call upon your purity now.
    You stand for fertility, for love, for motherhood.
    Lend to me your aid this day.

11. Center and ground again, then empower the moonstone with your hopes and positive dreams for your pregnancy. Visualize yourself pregnant, full of life, healthy, joyful, and in harmony with the Divine. Allow these positive emotions to flow into the moonstone. If fears or trepidations arise in your heart and spirit while you are empowering the stone, acknowledge them, but allow them to flow away into the earth to which you are grounded instead of into the stone.

12. When you feel the stone has been empowered enough, place it on the lavender at the base of the candle. Sit or stand back and bask in the feelings of being loved and in harmony with the Goddess, or the hopes and pride you feel regarding the step you are taking.

13. Allow the candle to burn down completely before gathering up the lavender and the moonstone and placing them in the center of the square of cloth. If you so desire, you may include the

candle stub in the cloth as well once it has cooled down. Gather up the corners of the cloth and wrap the yarn or floss around the cloth, fastening it to create a small sachet. Tie it shut with three knots, visualizing your journey into pregnancy being blessed with each knot.

14. Thank the Goddess for her blessings in your own words. Release the elements, if you invoked them, and close your circle with your usual ritual closing, or if you have chosen to work in sacred space, simply say something like, *I depart in peace. Blessed be.*

15. Place the sachet on your pregnancy shrine or your altar.

Ritual for Enhanced Fertility

If you've been trying to get pregnant and haven't yet succeeded, try this ritual to help enhance your fertility. As always, speak with your medical professional if you are concerned about the situation, and follow up your magical work with action in the real world.

This ritual uses the figure known as the Venus of Willendorf as a fertility symbol upon which to focus and from whom to draw sympathetic magic. The Venus of Willendorf is a Paleolithic statuette of an idealized female figure found near Willendorf, Austria. It's made of limestone and tinted with red ochre, and measures approximately 4⅜" high. This female figure has exaggerated breasts, abdomen, and vulva, with tiny arms and no recognizable

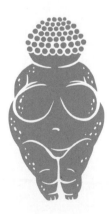

face, prompting many to draw a connection between her and the concept of the universal Earth Mother. You may make a copy of this specific figure, or use it as inspiration to design your own, guided by your intuition during the process.

If you wish, listen to music during this ritual. Choose something that makes you think of fertility. You may also burn incense and a candle; choose a scent and a color that also evoke fertility for you.

Make sure the type of clay you get is self-hardening, also known as air-drying, which does not require baking to set. Work on a surface that is flat, and cover your surface with plastic or newspaper to protect it from the clay.

YOU WILL NEED

- ❖ Candle with candleholder (optional)
- ❖ Incense with censer (optional)
- ❖ Matches or a lighter (optional)
- ❖ Plastic or newspaper to protect your work surface
- ❖ Self-hardening clay (about the size of your fist), color of your choice
- ❖ 1 tablespoon dried red clover
- ❖ Reference picture of the Venus of Willendorf (optional)
- ❖ 1 malachite stone (about $1/2$" in diameter, or smaller)
- ❖ Tools to work the clay (needle, chopstick, stylus, and so on)
- ❖ Paint for the dried clay (optional)

DIRECTIONS

1. Create sacred space as per your usual practice.

2. If you have chosen to use a candle and/or incense, light them now.

3. Invoke the Goddess with these or similar words:

   Great Goddess,
   Giver of fruitfulness and life,

> *Queen of fertility and abundance,*
> *Be with me now as I create this image.*
> *Let it draw physical fertility to me*
> *And allow me to conceive a child.*
> *Welcome, Queen of Fertility.*

4. Take the clay and begin to knead it, in order to soften it. As you knead, visualize the clay glowing with fertile energy. Once it is soft, flatten it out with your hands.

5. Pick up the red clover in your hands and hold it in your cupped palm. Breathe onto it three times, visualizing your breath infusing it with life.

6. Sprinkle the clover evenly over the flattened clay. Roll up the clay, then form it into a ball. Knead it again to distribute the clover throughout the clay.

7. Begin to form the clay into a shape approximating that of the Venus of Willendorf. It is not necessary (or indeed, important) to make an exact replica; the Venus of Willendorf is serving as inspiration for your own fertility goddess figure.

8. When you have a rough approximation of what you want your fertility goddess to look like, carefully hollow out an opening in her abdomen. Press the malachite stone into that opening. If you wish, you can then carefully cover it by smoothing the clay to the sides over the stone. Alternatively, if you wish to leave the malachite showing, smooth only a bit of clay over the edges of the stone to help keep it in place.

9. Finish smoothing and shaping the fertility goddess as you desire. Add details with tools such as a knitting needle, a chopstick, a stylus, or a ballpoint pen whose ink has dried up.

10. Thank the Goddess in your own words for her presence and her blessing. Take down your sacred space as per your usual practice.

11. Leave the fertility goddess statue in a safe place to dry. If your fertility figure has very thick areas, the clay may need more time to dry out properly. Turn it at some point so that it dries evenly.

12. When dry, you may paint your fertility figure or leave it as it is. (Check the packaging of the clay for suggestions regarding what kind of paint to use.)

13. Place the figure on your pregnancy shrine. Thank the Goddess again for her presence and energy.

Meditation on Becoming Pregnant

Meditation can be a valuable method of exploring your feelings about a subject and of allowing yourself the opportunity to listen to your emotions in an uninterrupted, welcoming fashion. This meditation is very simple and can help you explore your feelings about your choice to become pregnant or the news that you are pregnant.

DIRECTIONS

1. Create sacred space as per your usual practice. This meditation does not require a circle; sacred space is fine. If you use incense or music as a regular aid to meditation, you may do so for this meditation as well.

2. Sit on the floor or in a chair and close your eyes. Breathe deeply a few times. As you inhale, draw calm into your body; as you exhale, release tension.

3. When you feel relaxed, visualize the form of a pregnant woman. What feelings arise in you?

4. Consider the word *pregnant*. What is your emotional response to this word?

5. When you are finished meditating, note down your responses in your magical journal or Book of Shadows. (See Chapter 6 for ideas for creating a spiritual pregnancy journal.) Take time to look at the emotional responses you have experienced. You may wish to write a response to them.

Chapter 2

Exploring the Universal Mother

Like any other event in life, pregnancy and birthing have a multitude of customs attached to them. In Western culture many of the customs associated directly with labor and the delivery of a child have been stripped away, and as a result the experience has been somewhat diminished, brought down to only the physical process. By looking to other cultures you can see that customs both ancient and modern reflect the spiritual aspects of the act, and by considering them you can perhaps better encompass the spiritual dimension of your own pregnancy.

Traditionally, labor and birth were considered women's mysteries, and this is still true in some cultures. Women are there to aid, support, and surround the laboring woman; men either are not allowed or choose to be elsewhere, based on the belief that their presence would somehow diminish their masculinity or adversely affect the delivery and resulting child. Childbirth, like other women's mysteries, allows a connection to be made between the laboring woman and all her female ancestors, as well as her ultimate ancestor and mother, the Goddess.

Traditions and Folk Wisdom Surrounding Pregnancy

The cultural traditions and folk beliefs surrounding pregnancy aren't necessarily based in provable fact. Instead, they are often drawn from making observations about an act or situation and extrapolating those observations to the pregnant woman. This is an illustration of the sympathetic principle, or the concept of "like is drawn to like."

The sympathetic principle is perhaps the most common foundation for ritual and spellwork. A similarity is observed between two disparate objects or actions, and a link is thus made between the two. This correspondence is seen to be a medium through which one thing may be affected by influencing the other. This is the basis for many customs throughout the world and for the system of correspondences so often used in ritual and spells. The sympathetic principle also functions through imitative action (for example, if a woman wishes to become pregnant, she may ritually enact the physical behavior of pregnancy, then labor and delivery, and finally caring for an infant) and sympathetic participation in an act (for example, having a woman who is attempting to bring on labor be present at the childbed of another woman delivering her baby). Also on the principle of "like attracts like," having women who have successfully carried and delivered a baby at the childbed of a first-time mother is thought to lend success to the laboring woman.

Customs Associated with Gestation

In some cultures, a pregnant woman is seen as unwell; in others, she is seen as the pinnacle of health and life.

In her book *Childbirth Wisdom: From the World's Oldest Societies*, Judith Goldsmith says, "Pregnancy does not signal an abrupt change for women in tribal societies. They take it in their stride, going on with their everyday activities even to the last moments of birth." In fact, lethargy is seen as a possible way to have a listless baby; maintaining physical activity during pregnancy keeps the baby vital and energetic. In contrast, Western women are encouraged to take time off before pregnancy and to be careful regarding their physical activity.

The diet of the gestating mother depends on the culture and geographical location, but there are some common beliefs. For example, pregnant women are often warned to avoid hot, bitter, or spicy foods, as they are thought to adversely affect the development of the fetus. In many cultures they are also urged to avoid sweets and milk, as it is sometimes believed that these can cause the fetus to grow too large, making delivery more difficult.

In China, women are urged to eat "cold" foods to balance the "hot" condition of pregnancy. Cold and hot in this instance refer to the two polarities of chi, or life energy, in Chinese philosophy, referred to as yin and yang energies. Yin and yang are polarity points that may be expressed as negative and positive (as in the polarity of a magnet, not a value). Yin is perceived as being cool, feminine, receptive energy, whereas yang is perceived as being warm, masculine, active energy. These two points are opposing but complementary, meaning that they must continually work together in order to maintain a balance. Life energy is in constant motion, and a balance is sought by introducing yin energy where there is too much yang, and vice versa.

Some cultures believe that the specific food cravings the mother experiences are expressions of the desires of the child she carries. In Western culture, these cravings are often explained as the pregnant body requiring certain nutrients found in the desired food. Other food-associated customs include a belief found in both Filipino and some other Asian cultures that eating foods such as squid renders the womb tenacious (the tentacular nature of the creature can symbolically hold the baby back and make labor difficult), and the Turkish belief that pregnant women should eat foods that are round, such as grapes and quince, to help develop and protect the pregnancy.

Pregnant women are also commonly cautioned to avoid funerals and graveyards, for fear that spirits of the dead may attempt to seize the baby's life for their own in order to be reborn. The association of death is in general something pregnant women avoid, in an attempt to defend the life energy of their baby. Another widespread association is that of negative emotion damaging the baby in some way. Pregnant women are therefore counseled to avoid anger and distress.

Another cross-cultural bit of folk wisdom is the caution with which pregnant women are advised to handle sharp objects such as knives and scissors. If a sharp-bladed object is held pointing to the fetus, or left on the bed, it is thought that the fetus may develop a cleft palate or lip.

Polynesian women are encouraged to make peace with people they have wronged, have misunderstandings with, or hold grudges against. This is thought to ease labor and delivery by removing obstacles.

Customs Associated with Labor

Unlike Western medicine, which expects women to lie down during their labor, in many tribal societies walking or other physical activity is encouraged to help the baby be born. Perhaps because of this, Goldsmith notes that, in general, tribal deliveries are shorter than modern Western births.

The laboring woman is often accompanied by women who have successfully given birth, an example of associating sympathetic activity. A common cross-cultural belief is that the laboring woman must not wear any necklaces, as the umbilical cord may wrap around the baby's neck. Similarly, in Turkey as in other countries, the laboring woman's hair is unbound and allowed to flow freely in order to remove any obstacles that may be holding the baby back. Likewise, doors and windows may be opened so that the baby will not be held back by any associated symbols.

Customs Associated with Delivery

Unlike in Western culture, the actual delivery in many tribal cultures is witnessed by trusted friends and family, not strangers.

Physical positions for delivery vary from culture to culture, but common positions include sitting with the knees drawn up to the chest, kneeling, or squatting (usually supported by a bar or rope, sometimes called a birthing rope, because this position is physically demanding). Lying down on one's back to give birth is rare in tribal cultures, for this position is seen as lazy and does not encourage the child to move. If lying down is done, it is usually done on the side. In the past in Europe, the birthing chair was often used. The birthing chair was a low chair with a horseshoe-shaped seat, with an open front and middle to allow the birth attendant to catch the baby. In ancient Egypt, women giving birth squatted on two bricks, raising them farther off the floor to facilitate catching the newborn.

Postbirth Customs

Many cultures also have customs related to postbirth events. For instance, in China it was the father's responsibility to give the newborn its first bath. In several cultures the new mother goes through a period of low exposure to water for two to four weeks after delivery, limiting her to sponge baths.

Beliefs and customs involving the placenta vary, but most cultures respect it as being tied spiritually to the baby. Actions vary, from the placenta being buried near the child's home for protection, sometimes with a tree planted over it to help root the child in their new life and to help provide stability for them, to the mother cooking and eating the placenta to help nourish her in the demanding first weeks of her new role. In modern North America, the placenta is usually disposed of, but the stump of the umbilical cord is sometimes kept once it falls off.

Childbirth As a Rite of Passage

Rite of passage is a term describing the transition from one position within society to another, whereby an individual's social status is changed in some fashion. According to ethnographer Arnold van Gennep, a rite of passage has three formal stages:

1. **Separation, or the preliminal stage.** In this stage, the individual is socially and emotionally uprooted from her present life and the role she has played within society, and, as a consequence, spiritually uprooted as well. This first stage incorporates reflection and the beginning of knowledge acquisition in preparation for the new role.

2. **Transformation, or the liminal stage.** In this second stage, the individual is in a liminal state, not belonging to the old position and not yet part of the new position.

3. **Reincorporation, or the postliminal stage.** In this third and final stage, the individual is absorbed into the community in the new role.

Due to a rite of passage involving a threshold, the individual undergoing the rite does not exist in one world, nor in the other; instead, the individual is of both and neither simultaneously. This places you in the curious position of not belonging but of still having a unique perspective into both worlds. This is a time outside of time and a place of great spiritual wisdom and secret knowledge, for you occupy a place and moment usually sacred to priests and priestesses, the instruments of the gods. The secret knowledge gained during a rite of passage is not necessarily accessible afterward. It is, however, encoded in your soul, a part of you, and your subconscious can draw upon it. It will affect you for the rest of your life even though you may not consciously remember it on a day-to-day basis.

Spiritually, a rite of passage allows a connection to the Divine as the threshold is crossed. Connecting with the Goddess during the process of childbirth is not something you have to consciously do or attempt to do. This connection forms naturally as you participate in the sympathetic act of giving birth, just as the Goddess has done thousands of times, and as millions of women have done since the dawn of time.

The rite of passage encoded in pregnancy and childbirth is not only a rite of passage for the woman involved, but also for the child. During the pregnancy (particularly conception and gestation, and often birthing as well) the main focus is usually on the experience of the expectant mother, and only marginally on that of the child in formation. This is unfair to the child, whose experience is mostly a mystery to us but still spiritually valid. After delivery, the focus tends to switch to the child as physical and tangible evidence of the rite of passage, which is in turn moderately unfair to the mother, who must still reintegrate into regular, everyday life. Rituals such as Wiccanings, namings, baby blessings, and baptisms all focus on welcoming and integrating the infant into the community, but there exists little formal support for the mother as she attempts to function within her new social position.

It is important to remember that the immense spiritual transition experienced by both mother and child is to be celebrated and supported. The new infant is in itself a change, but the mother also transforms, both within herself and within her community. Working throughout your pregnancy with awareness of this transition will help prepare you for the experience; if you have a partner, the process will be a pivotal transition for you both, and keeping this awareness in your minds and hearts will help you support each other with love.

Chapter 3

Embodying the Goddess

The twentieth century saw the rise in popularity of a concept known as the triple goddess, a triad-natured female deity. The three aspects encompassed youth, adulthood, and the senior years, referred to respectively as the Maiden, the Mother, and the Crone. This concept was then retroactively applied to groups of goddesses throughout history and various cultures.

In theory, the triple goddess is an attractive grouping. Threes tend to be sacred in Western culture, and the idea of an all-inclusive goddess format like this makes sure no one is left out. However, it's equally confusing at times, because there are some goddesses that are difficult to classify. Does one assign a goddess to a certain aspect because she has associations in common with that aspect? Does one classify a goddess according to her portrayed age?

This chapter will explore these aspects of the Goddess and how they relate to motherhood and pregnancy. We'll also look at some deities associated with motherhood and pregnancy and reflect on how you can work with them and draw inspiration from them during your pregnancy.

Exploring the Triple Goddess

The triple-aspect concept is a purely human construct, used to help us organize our thoughts. One such classification is obvious: The Mother aspect of the Goddess is the one most clearly associated with pregnancy and motherhood. Goddesses of childbirth tend to also be Mother goddesses, which makes a certain amount of sense, although it is interesting to note that there are also selections of various cultural Maiden and Crone aspects who oversee pregnancy and childbirth. The Crone is experienced, has reached a point where she possibly has had several pregnancies herself, and has delivered others. The association of the Maiden aspect with pregnancy and childbirth is slightly more complex. In our modern society, we tend to assume that the term *maiden* means "virgin," or sexually uninitiated, which can confuse contemporary women who expect a goddess associated with pregnancy or childbirth to have at least some firsthand experience of the process. In fact, the Maiden aspect refers more to the idea of a free young woman, beholden to no one and in control of her own life and destiny. Artemis of Greek myth is one such virgin figure who defends and protects women in childbirth. In some versions of her myth she is said to have assisted her mother, Leto, with the delivery of her twin brother, Apollo.

These three separate aspects of the Goddess can be problematic when you're trying to figure out how you fit in. Each aspect possesses several levels and depths of meaning. Often, however, these multiple meanings and associations become overshadowed by the stereotype associated with the aspect.

Part of the mystery of the Goddess is that the three aspects are in fact defined by one another. The Mother is a mother as compared to the Crone and the Maiden; the Maiden is a younger woman as compared to the two older aspects. There are no clear-cut divisions between these aspects either. One does not cease being a Maiden at a defined moment or with a specific act. It can be argued that every woman holds all three aspects within herself, with one simply more prominent at any given time. Every woman's personality and spirit reflect all three aspects simultaneously, and she can call upon any aspect to help her understand a situation or challenge.

None of these aspects are "good" or "bad." Each aspect encompasses both dark and light. For example, the Mother teaches us to nurture, but an overabundance of nurturing leads to smothering a child's independence as the mother clings. The natural love of a mother can turn to anger and resentment under certain conditions.

Remember: The triple aspect of the Goddess is a relatively modern concept, applied to the goddesses of other cultures in general by neo-pagans. It is by no means a universal formula.

The Aspects of the Goddess

While you are close to the Goddess at every moment of your life, somehow it can be easier to sense it while pregnant. While carrying a child, you become very aware of the rhythm of the life force as it flows around and through you. While your obvious affinity may be to the Mother aspect, the aspects of Maiden and Crone also influence your spiritual transformation.

The Maiden

Youth, potential, purity, innocence, creativity, imagination—these are the Maiden's traditional associations. The Maiden represents the ability to learn, the thirst for knowledge, and the freedom to experience life in all its forms. In physical expression, the term *maiden* is sometimes applied to a young woman whose menses has not yet begun. Menses is indicative of the body's physical readiness to reproduce. In today's society, physical readiness does not indicate emotional or social readiness. These latter two classifications are indeed more of what determine our preparedness or state of readiness to conceive, bear, and nurture a child.

The aspect of the Maiden encompasses the freedom associated with childhood and adolescence. Purity is the stereotypical association with this aspect—often physical purity. The Maiden is not defined by her abstinence from sexual activity, however, nor is she defined by a lack of sexual experience or initiation. Instead, the Maiden is characterized by several different freedoms:

❖ **FREEDOM FROM SOCIAL STRUCTURES:** The Maiden is unaffected by the expectations and directives of society. She remains free to do what she desires, functioning apart from social pressure and peer influence. She is self-defined and subservient to no one.

❖ **FREEDOM FROM IMPOSED RESPONSIBILITY:** Beholden to no one but herself, the Maiden makes her own decisions and applies her energies to the areas and issues where she feels drawn to apply them. Self-motivated, she works where she feels she is needed and where her efforts will yield both personal and universal benefit.

❖ **FREEDOM FROM EXPECTATIONS:** With no imposed roles, the Maiden is free to define her own successes and failures.

❖ **FREEDOM FROM SEXUAL ROLES:** The Maiden doesn't play power games when it comes to sex and relationships. Functioning without social expectations, she refuses to be defined by sexual experience and sexual activity. This also means that the Lover is part of this aspect, for the Maiden as Lover shares herself freely and without expectation with her partners. The term *virgin* originally meant a woman not married or otherwise associated legally with a man, or without the responsibility of a family. This also implies a self-sufficient woman, as well as those still considered part of her father's family. When taken in this respect, the Maiden certainly indicates an aspect fully defined by herself and no other.

How long does the Maiden aspect last? As stated before, at no time does any one aspect cease to exist in an individual. Rather, there are times in our life when one aspect flows to the forefront and the others recede slightly, still offering their wisdom and energy, simply not to the same intensity as they have done at other times.

The Mother

Bounty, fertility, nurturing, life-giving—all these are standard associations with the Mother aspect of the Goddess. Associated with the earth itself, with the full moon, and with the sea, the Mother is often the default image of the Goddess. She is the universal mother, the womb who brings forth all life, the provider, and the comforter.

It is odd that such an all-encompassing aspect is, in fact, poorly defined. The term *mother* carries with it so many inferences and associations that it is all too easy to simply use it and expect everyone to understand what it entails. The Mother is perhaps the vaguest aspect of the Goddess, for all her universal recognition.

The Mother is ripe sexuality and fertility of both body and fields. Her crops are the young of humankind and animals, the birds of the air, and the denizens of the seas, as well as the green of the fields. She is also darkness: the warm wet darkness of the womb, the night from which all things emerge. She is that darkness of fresh, rich earth, from which life can spring. The Mother teaches you that your body is sacred, and how to care for it and for others, and how to nurture and nourish.

The Mother has a difficult role to play. It is easy enough to nurture and love, but a mother must also step back and allow her children to fall down, to be hurt, and to make mistakes. Mothering is not held exclusive to human children either: We nurture and care for the people around us, the plants and trees, our pets and animal companions. How we express the aspect of the Mother as she manifests within us varies from person to person. The Mother is:

❖ **CREATOR:** The Mother is the creator aspect of the triple goddess. Her capacity for bringing forth life lends her this association. The Mother's fruitfulness and fertility make her the ideal aspect upon whom to call if you are in search of energy with which to bring forth any kind of project. The creator aspect is not the same as a muse; while the Creator Mother can inspire, she is the embodiment of the act of creation rather than the impetus that begins the process.

❖ **WARRIOR:** The Mother is also a warrior, the one who rises to meet threats and challenges, who defends her young. This aspect of the Goddess is often perceived as violent, and while she does possess the capacity for violence if the situation requires it, the Warrior Mother is first and foremost a defender.

❖ **QUEEN:** The Mother aspect is the enthroned queen, she who rules over humanity and all living things. The Goddess Queen is traditionally an aspect of the awareness of, and spirit of, the land, and the one who bestows sovereignty upon a ruler. Likewise, she is the queen of the earth itself, she who rules every living thing. The role of a queen is to care for her people, to inspire them, to be a figure of love and respect. The Mother aspect fills this role: regal, stately, and Goddess imperial. The Empress card from the tarot's Major Arcana embodies the concept of Queen Mother.

The Crone

The Crone is the wisewoman, the grandmother, the elder who teaches and passes on her valuable experience to those younger than she is. She is often associated with healing, for her age gives her the advantage of having encountered illness and injury in her community, and the knowledge of how to deal successfully with both. Often, a woman is thought to begin her transition into the realm of the Crone with the onset of menopause, which occurs on average around the age of fifty-one. The time of the Crone is an honorable stage of life, and one to be embraced with as much joy and respect as the two earlier stages of Maiden and Mother. The Crone is associated with:

❖ **TEACHING:** The Crone is a teacher, one who passes on knowledge and information. Because she has lived so long and seen so much, the Crone is also the aspect of the Goddess who is associated with secrets and the art of divination. The Crone teaches us the fullness of life, how to look back and embrace the totality of our experiences. She teaches us to honor the past, and our achievements, and also to be humble about them.

❖ **WISDOM:** One of the Crone's main associations is that of wisewoman. Traditionally, a wisewoman was attached to a village or region, an accessible individual who could be consulted about a variety of life problems. She is knowledgeable in the ways of nature and can often recommend a simple herb or combination of herbs to help someone who is ailing, or serve as a counselor. She can conduct rites of passage, pass along history, facilitate births and funerals, and perform small works of folk magic. The wisewoman is generally an older woman, and by virtue of her experience and private study, she can dispense information to those who ask for it. In a mystic sense, the wisewoman is one who is in touch with the mysteries of nature and of spirit, and by working with her one may uncover deep truths within oneself and attune to the rhythms of life.

❖ **SACRIFICE:** The Crone shows us how to pare away those things that hold us back, slow us down, or lessen us in some way. She shows us how to release the baggage we have thought necessary for so many years and how to carry on again after we have done so. The Crone does not demand sacrifice of us; it is simply a part of living. "Sacrifice is inherent in life, in constant change that brings constant losses," says Starhawk. Through these sacrifices, however, we come closer and closer to our essence, our pure self, while also creating the opportunity for new things in our lives.

❖ **DEATH:** Often, the Crone is associated with death and endings, just as the Maiden is associated with beginnings. Because the Crone is associated with the elderly, who are traditionally closest to the point of physical death in the life cycle, she is often stereotyped as the bringer of death. This is a regretful shame, because in today's society the senior population lives so much longer than ever before, and age does not immediately equal death. This population contains much knowledge, experience, and value, and to automatically parallel it with the concept of death is to ignore the richness of life contained within those aggregated years. The Crone is not the final moment of life; she is the last third of the full life experience.

It is true that the aspect of the Goddess who is associated with those who die is the Crone, but this is also due to the fact that it is often the elders of a society who sit with a dying individual and who traditionally prepare a body for burial. Those same elders are the ones who help babies to be born. Death is simply a passage from one state of being to another, much like birth; and at each, someone must take the newly transited soul into her arms for comfort and security. So the Crone is associated with endings, as the Maiden is associated with beginnings. It is important, however, to remember that death is not an ending, nor are all endings final, for life moves in a cycle, and an ending is simply a beginning in a different form. Nor is the Crone the one who deals out death; death is simply a natural occurrence.

The Crone is the one who takes your hand as you die, to ease your transition.

The Crone is also associated with transformation, the step from life through death to what lies beyond. The Crone is acceptance, too, and rest. She is honest evaluation. She is truth, and she is the time between activity and new beginnings, where we pause to take in our bearings and to gather our strength for the coming action.

Working with Goddesses While Pregnant

You may already have an established relationship with a goddess who is connected in some way with pregnancy or childbirth. If you do, you may wish to begin focusing on that particular aspect if you have not previously worked with it.

In a sense, all goddesses are echoes of the Great Goddess, and as such they are all in some way connected to the life-giving energy contained within the Divine Feminine. However, some goddesses have a stronger or clearer connection to that aspect of the Divine Feminine, and it can be easier to work with a goddess whose main function is related to pregnancy or motherhood in some way.

You should begin a relationship with a pregnancy-associated goddess near the start of your pregnancy and work with her throughout, in order to attune to her and her energies. In this way, you will have had a lot of time to develop your relationship with her and be better able to work with her during your labor and birthing, a stressful time when you will want as much help as possible.

The choosing of a goddess with whom to work throughout your pregnancy isn't done by flipping through these pages and picking one at random. Like choosing a roommate, this requires complementary personalities and a willingness to cooperate. Think about the cultures to which you are drawn, or the cultures from which your ancestors came. Read up on these goddesses in books of mythology, in encyclopedias, or in books devoted to them. The energy you will be working with will affect you deeply, as working with deity energy always does.

The following sections include less familiar goddesses as well as popular ones. However, there exists less documentation on some of them and therefore the information here may be less detailed than you would like. You should research on your own and meditate upon these goddesses in order to find the best match for you during your pregnancy. Also later in this chapter, there is a ritual to help you harmonize with the Mother Goddess, which may be adapted to help you work with a specific cultural manifestation of the Mother Goddess by using symbols and titles specific to your chosen goddess.

Here are some suggestions to help you meditate on a specific mother goddess:

❖ Meditate on a symbol associated with her: for example, Demeter with a sheaf of grain, Hera with a pomegranate or cow, Isis with wings or an ankh, and so forth.

❖ Meditate on a visual depiction of the goddess: a portrait, an ancient cultural statue or carving, or a modern interpretation in statue or picture form.

❖ Imagine meeting the goddess in a place where you feel safe. If you have an established meditation landscape, do it there.

Otherwise, imagine yourself in a place in which the goddess would be comfortable, perhaps a culturally appropriate temple. Speak with the goddess about how you feel, and ask her if she would be willing to help you, or if she has any advice for you.

❖ Paint or draw a picture while thinking about the goddess.

Great Mother Goddesses

Generally, the goddess you'll be working with will be a Mother aspect. This makes perfect sense. If the goddess with whom you wish to work is of another aspect, look at the associations with that aspect and think about how they correspond to your pregnancy. A goddess of the Maiden aspect may have valuable things to teach you about maintaining your sense of individuality; a Crone aspect may have wisdom about the process of birthing and healing to pass on to you.

As you read through the following references, you may be struck by certain commonalities such as grain, cattle, and pomegranates. These symbols seem to come up again and again in the iconography of mother goddesses. Try meditating on each of them, and see what associations they evoke from you. Perhaps add a depiction of one or more to your pregnancy shrine. Pomegranates are easy to come by in markets: Try eating a few of the seeds while performing a ritual or as you meditate on the cycle of life and the importance of fertility within that cycle. Don't forget to journal your responses.

Isis

Perhaps the most famous of goddesses, Isis is a deity of the Egyptian pantheon who absorbed many of the older goddesses and their fields of provenance. Two of her strongest associations are fertility and motherhood, making her an ideal goddess with whom to work during pregnancy and afterward. Isis is also an excellent deity to call on if you are having difficulty conceiving, for she conceived her son after magically bringing her husband back from the dead. This son is Horus, the Egyptian god associated with humankind. Isis is thus associated with motherhood in general, so working with her throughout your pregnancy will help attune you to the energy of the Mother aspect of the Goddess.

Isis's worship absorbed many of Hathor's associations (see later section in this chapter: Deities Associated with Pregnancy and Birth) as her popularity grew. Her many epithets point to the strong association she held in the minds of the Egyptian people regarding her connections to fertility: She Who Gives Birth to Heaven and Earth; Mother of the Gods; Lady of Green Crops; and Goddess of Fertility, Nature, and Motherhood.

Cybele

Also known as Kybele and Magna Mater (literally the "great mother"), Cybele is of Phrygian origin, in the Asia Minor area. Her original association was with the earth, the first fertile progenitor of life. Her Greek cognate is Rhea. Cybele is associated with caves, a physical parallel to the depths of the earth from where life emerges. Cybele is also connected to wild animals, nature, mountains, and fertility. Her worship involved wild music, dancing, and singing, often with orgiastic and violent rites, so be cautious if you work with her, for those who traditionally served her sometimes got carried away. You may find yourself dealing with very marked emotional swings and with impassioned emotional responses to situations and incidents during your pregnancy.

Lions are one of Cybele's animals, and she is often portrayed in a chariot being pulled by two of them.

Demeter

Demeter is the Greek goddess of grain and fertility. Her name means "grain mother." Demeter is the mother of Persephone, the maiden who was taken to the underworld by Hades to be his bride. Demeter searched the earth for her daughter, allowing her responsibility to maintain the growth and production of crops to slip away. As a result, the growth cycle came to a halt. When Persephone could not be found, Demeter gave way to her grief. As she mourned, all green and growing things withered away. When Persephone was eventually found and reunited with her mother, the land reflected Demeter's joy, and gave forth life again. Persephone had eaten a few pomegranate seeds while in the underworld, and as a result was ordered to spend one month with Hades in the underworld for each seed she had consumed. When Persephone descends into the underworld each year, Demeter mourns anew, and the land also mourns. This myth is an explanation of the cycle of life: life and production, then death, or a fallow period, or what are often simply sorted into a summer and winter season. Persephone herself is often correlated with spring and the return of life.

Demeter's gift to humankind was grain, the cultivating of which differentiated them from animals. Thus Demeter is indirectly associated with agriculture and civilization as well. She is often accompanied by harvest imagery such as sheaves or baskets of grain, sickles and scythes, ploughs, fruit and vegetables, and garlands or wreaths of wheat ears.

The sow is one of the animals directly associated with Demeter. Horses are also considered her animals, and Demeter is sometimes portrayed with a mare's head in older Greek art. Poppies and pomegranates, as symbols of life and death, are also associated with Demeter.

Demeter's Roman cognate is Ceres. Persephone's Roman cognate is Proserpine.

Hera

The Greek goddess of marriage and wives, Hera was the consort of Zeus, although her existence goes further back in history. Her main areas of association are birth and death, and as a protector of women in general. Later myths have her attempting to stop various births, seemingly for jealous reasons (often because the infant had been sired by her consort Zeus); drawing from this, Hera may be called upon to keep a pregnancy safe and secure until the natural time for birth has come. When one examines the later myths that portray Hera as a jealous, uptight wife who defends the rights of the wife in marriage, she would seem to be a mother goddess associated mainly with children born of a sanctioned marriage. Earlier pre-Zeus versions of these myths likely portrayed her as a very different goddess; it is theorized that the Hera mythology was reinterpreted with the arrival of the Zeus-based worship, reducing Hera to a conquered goddess married to the main god of a new pantheon in order to legitimize him. It is important to remember, however, that the union of a god and goddess is often a symbol for the affirmation of the life-creating principle, the physical union of male and female energies. The *hieros gamos*, "the sacred marriage," is a fertility rite conducted in several cultures that often incorporates the actual sexual act in order to stimulate fertile energies in the land or people. One myth suggests that Hera's virginity is restored annually when the goddess bathes in the spring of Canathus. This suggests that the rite or union is performed regularly in order to ensure that the fertility of the land is continued, with the virgin Hera offering the potential contained within her physical body as a sacrifice. In her status with Zeus, Hera is very much a consort and queen, two other facets associated with the Mother aspect of the Goddess.

However, there exists a myth that tells of Hera bringing forth children on her own without the involvement of Zeus or any other male figure, either by sitting on the ground and beating the earth with her hand or by eating lettuce, a vegetable associated with lactation (and, curiously, impotence for men). Both these techniques are interesting for their earth associations—the earth is, of course, a source of life and sustenance, a symbol of abundance and fertility in its own right. Beating the earth is a physical working of it, akin to the toil and labor put in by agricultural workers. Lettuce is a low-growing vegetable pulled directly from the earth, the leaves of which are broad, which evokes images of plates or bowls (feminine symbols), and green, a color associated with abundance and fertility for its predominance in the natural world.

Hera is strongly associated with cattle; indeed, one of the most common epithets applied to her is Cow-Eyed. *Hera* translates to "lady." Her chariot is said to be pulled by peacocks, and her favorite bird is the cuckoo. The fruit she is most often depicted with is the pomegranate.

Interestingly enough, Hera is the mother of Eileithyia, the Greek goddess of childbirth.

Gaea

Gaea (also spelled Gaia) is the prototypical mother goddess, and her name is often given to our planet as a sign of our appreciation for Earth's bounty and life-giving properties. She is sometimes known as Ge. In the "Homeric Hymn 30 to Gaia" Homer says:

> To Gaia (Earth) the Mother of All. I will sing of well-founded Gaia (Earth), mother of all, eldest of all beings. She feeds all the creatures that are in the worlds, all that go upon the goodly land, and all that are in the paths of the seas, and all that fly: all these are fed of her store. Through you, O queen, men are blessed in their children and blessed in their harvests, and to you it belongs to give means of life to mortal men and to take it away.

In the "Orphic Hymn 26 to Ge" Orpheus says of her:

> O mother Gaia, of Gods and men the source, endured with fertile, all-destroying force; all-parent, bounding, whose prolific powers produce a store of beauteous fruits and flowers. All-various maid, the immortal world's strong base, eternal, blessed, crowned with every grace; from whose wide womb as from an endless root, fruits many-formed, mature, and grateful shoot. Deep-bosomed, blessed, pleased with grassy plains, sweet to the smell, and with prolific rains. All-flowery Daimon, centre of the world, around thy orb the beauteous stars are hurled with rapid whirl, eternal and divine, whose frames with matchless skill and wisdom shine. Come, blessed Goddess, listen to my prayer, and make increase of fruits thy constant care; with fertile seasons (*horai*) in thy train draw near, and with propitious mind thy suppliants hear.

Both these examples point to the reverence paid to Gaea for her power over humans, animals, and vegetation. The turn of the seasons is associated with Gaea, as are seeds and roots, plants themselves, harvests, animals, and humankind. It was Gaea who created a new flower with which Hades lured Persephone into the underworld. And yet Gaea is also the compassionate goddess who often hears and answers the pleas of nymphs and women chased by gods, turning them into plants and trees to rescue them from unwanted attention. She also serves as the nursemaid to a few other gods and heroes.

Gaea was the original deity power behind the oracle at Delphi. The concept of prophecy, guidance, and answers originating from the mysterious depths of the earth parallels the potential encompassed by the newborn infant emerging from the fertile darkness. Oaths sworn in the name of Gaea were considered extremely binding, underlining the association of the earth with stability and permanence, and imbuing the oath sworn by the goddess of Earth with that same energy.

There are several different versions of Gaea's myths, but in one she is the daughter of Light and Day. In another she herself gave birth to the heavens (Uranus), the mountains, and the sea, and then with the heavens creates several other children, including the Titans. In another origin myth a serpent encircles an egg and squeezes it into two separate parts, which are Gaea (earth) and Uranus (sky).

Danu

Also known as Dana, Ana, and Anu, Danu is a pan-Celtic goddess, but mainly associated with Ireland. Her Welsh cognate is Dôn. She is the great mother goddess of the Irish people, the founder of the line of Tuatha Dé Danann (people of Danu), which includes many of the popularly known gods such as Brigid, Lugh, the Dagda, Lir, and so forth.

Danu is strongly associated with water, and indeed, her name may be associated with the proto-Celtic word meaning "flow," "fast," or "water." In fact, she appears to be more strongly associated with water than with land, an interesting divergence from the more customary earth association held by mother goddesses.

As is the case with most of the other Celtic deities, there exists little primary source reference to Danu. The collective unconscious is a strong force, however, and it has firmly assigned Danu the associations of fertility and abundance.

Ritual to Harmonize with the Mother Goddess

This ritual is designed to give you a place from which to start working with a specific mother goddess. This ritual is generic and addressed to the Mother Goddess, but if you wish to personalize it with the name and attributes of the specific mother goddess with whom you have chosen to work throughout your pregnancy, then replace the phrase *Mother Goddess* as desired. If you wish to further personalize the ritual to your chosen mother goddess, do a bit of research to find out what her favorite offerings are, and use them in addition to or instead of the milk and the rose. Offerings can include such things as flowers, scents, beverages, foods, art, and so forth.

This ritual uses the practice of libation, an offering of a beverage to a deity performed by pouring it out with ceremony. This is well suited to honoring the Mother Goddess for its thematic connection to flowing breast milk, a symbol of fertility and nurture. It may be repeated throughout your pregnancy when you feel moved to honor the Goddess.

The ritual may be done in a place of your choosing, so long as you feel comfortable there. You will need access to the outdoors for the libation offering, although this may be done after the ritual has been formally concluded. You can do this ritual with an altar or you can work with a simple setup of the supplies on the ground or a table in front of you. If you are lactose intolerant or sensitive to dairy products, the milk called for in the ritual can be replaced with soy or almond milk.

If you grow your own roses, use one of them no matter what the color. If you can find a wild white rose, use it; otherwise, one you buy at a florist will do. Do not strip the thorns off the rose you will use for this ritual. The thorns represent the pain and fortitude that comes with the beauty and strength of the Mother.

You may perform this ritual at any point during your pregnancy, and any number of times. You should perform it as early as possible, however, to maximize the time with which you attune to the Mother Goddess or the specific goddess with whom you wish to work.

YOU WILL NEED
- ❖ 1 white candle
- ❖ Candleholder
- ❖ Matches or a lighter
- ❖ A chalice or cup (silver or earthenware are ideal)
- ❖ Milk (poured into chalice)
- ❖ 1 white rose
- ❖ A small vase, preferably glass or crystal, with water in it (optional)

DIRECTIONS

1. Create sacred space according to your customary practice.

2. Invoke the Goddess as you light the candle:
   > *Mother,*
   > *Hear your daughter as she calls to you.*
   > *Descend to me, here in this sacred circle.*
   > *Share with me your love, your wisdom, and your strength.*
   > *Welcome, Mother, to my circle.*
   > *So may it be.*

3. Lift the chalice. Say:
   > *Mother Goddess, I honor you.*
   > *You bring life to the world.*
   > *Your milk nourishes us.*
   > *Walk with me throughout this pregnancy.*
   > *Grant me insight, patience, and serenity.*
   > *Yours is the life of the mother, as is the life of the child.*
   > *I open myself to your love and knowledge.*
   > *I welcome your presence.*
   > *Teach me; support me; love me.*
   > *Mother Goddess, I offer you the contents of this cup*
   > *In thanks for your everlasting care.*

4. Draw down the moon's energy into the chalice of milk, until the milk vibrates with the energy of the Mother Goddess. If you are unfamiliar with this technique, simply envision the energy of the moon pouring down from the luminary into the cup for as long as you feel it necessary. The cup may tingle in your hands, grow warm or cool; how you sense energy will determine your experience here. Visualize that energy being the nurturing energy of the Mother.

5. Take a sip of the milk you are offering to the Mother with aware-ness. As you swallow, visualize the energy contained within it spreading throughout your body, including to your child.

6. If you are outdoors, pour out the remaining milk onto the ground, or at the base of a tree. If you are indoors, place the cup on the altar again. Pick up the flower. Say:

    Mother, I offer you this white rose
    As a token of my love for you
    And in appreciation for your beauty and grace.
    Grant me the ability to see that beauty and grace in myself
    As my body changes and my child grows within me.
    Mother, blessed be.

7. Kiss the rose, then dip the rose into the milk on the ground or in the cup, just enough to get a drop or two on the petals. If you prefer, dip the tips of your fingers into the milk and sprinkle a few drops on the rose.

8. If you are outdoors, place the rose on the ground where you offered the libation of milk. If you are indoors, place the rose in the vase on the altar.

9. Thank the Goddess for her presence at the ritual:

    Mother, thank you for being with me here in my circle
    And for sharing this time with me.
    I know you will walk with me throughout my pregnancy
    And be there when I need your support and wisdom.
    Blessed Mother, hail and farewell.

10. Take down your sacred space, as per your usual practice. If you have worked indoors, take the cup of milk outside and pour it ceremoniously at the base of a tree or into a moving body of water.

11. You may choose to leave the rose on the place where you have made the libation of milk, to throw the rose into moving water, or to leave the rose on your altar for three days. If you keep the rose on your altar, after the third day remove it and carefully pull off the petals and dry them. Once dry, put them in a soft pouch or a small jar to use in pregnancy-related spells. You may leave them whole and use them one by one or crumble them and use a pinch in spells and rituals. Alternately, when the rose is dry, add it to your pregnancy shrine (see Chapter 1).

Deities Associated with Pregnancy and Birth

These goddesses are specifically associated with pregnancy and birth, as opposed to the previously mentioned deities, who are associated with motherhood in general. Note that the goddesses listed here are not necessarily associated with motherhood as well.

Goddesses of childbirth tend to also be Mother goddesses, which makes a certain amount of sense, although it is interesting to note that there are selections of Maiden and Crone aspects who oversee pregnancy and childbirth as well. As explored earlier in this chapter, the Maiden aspect refers more to the idea of a free young woman, beholden to no one and in control of her own life and destiny. (See the previous discussion on the three aspects of the Goddess.)

Arianrhod

Of Welsh myth, and appearing in the Mabinogion cycle, Arianrhod responded to the call of the king for a virgin footholder (a euphemism for a woman to represent the sovereignty of the land, whose relationship with the king lends his rule validity). Arianrhod affirmed that she was a virgin, but when the king tested her by asking her to step over his magician's rod, she gave birth to two infants: one called Dylan, who was part sea creature, and the other a preterm boy who became known as Lleu Llaw Gyffes (and who may be better known by his Irish cognate, Lugh). Arianrhod's precipitous initiation into motherhood is also represented by how her relationship with her second son plays out. She refuses to give him a name, present him with weapons, or allow him to marry a human woman, three actions reserved for the mother in her society. By withholding these things, Arianrhod demonstrates the power held by the mother over how a child is initiated into society.

Arianrhod thus can be called upon to help understand a mother's responsibilities and to come to terms with the transition from Maiden to Mother. Meditating on her story can also help you deal with emotions such as anger or denial about pregnancy, if yours is an unexpected one.

Brigid

One of the most popular goddesses among the neo-pagan crowd, the pan-Celtic goddess Brigid possesses strong associations with women and children. Her more specific associations include lactation, herd animals such as cows and sheep, and hearth and home. Brigid is also associated with the elements of fire and water, two elements that have close associations with pregnancy and birth. Fire is considered to be a symbol of life and fertility, and water is associated with transformation and life as well.

Brigid is honored at a February festival known as Imbolc, or Oimelc, which literally translates to "in the belly" or "milk of ewe." The direct correlation is to the season of lambing, but the fertile and nurturing associations apply very easily to women as well. These associations and areas of focus bring Brigid close to the hearts of pregnant and nursing women.

In some myths, Brigid personifies the maiden of spring who returns the spirit of life to the land, banishing the crone of winter and the seeming lifelessness of the earth.

Carmenta

Carmenta is a Roman goddess of childbirth and prophecy. She is one of the Camenae, a series of Roman goddesses of wells and springs. Here again you can see the association made between sacred water and childbirth. Carmenta was also a mother herself, making her an excellent goddess to work with for childbirth. Her association with prophecy is a logical one to embrace for childbirth, for at the birth of a child one naturally desires to know the future, both of the newborn and of the family into which they have been born. Carmenta is also a patron of midwives. Sometimes she is known as Carmentis. Some writers place her as one of the Fates, and indicate that offerings would be made to her not only for successful delivery, but also for some prophecy regarding the future of the infant.

The Carmentalia was her festival, taking place roughly two weeks into January, and celebrated mainly by women. The festival focused on Carmenta's ability to look into the past and future, an activity strongly associated with standing on a threshold between the two extreme points of life and death. Offerings of grain, fruit, and vegetables are best.

Eileithyia

Daughter of Hera, Eileithyia is the Greek goddess associated with childbirth. Her name translates to "childbearing" or sometimes "birth pain." Her Latin name is Ilithyia, and sometimes her Greek name is transliterated as Eleuthia.

Eileithyia possesses the capability of stopping and starting labor. Legend has it that by crossing her arms and legs she can prevent an infant from being born, holding the mother and child in an indeterminate state for as long as she chooses. For this reason, Eileithyia can be called upon to help deal with premature labor. As she is also associated with actual childbirth, she can also be called upon to bring labor to its natural conclusion if labor has gone on for some time with little progress.

The fig is associated with Eileithyia, which is said to be so connected because of the fruit's resemblance to a womb. The torch is also one of her symbols, for as midwife Eileithyia brings infants from darkness to light. She is often portrayed as veiled, which serves to highlight her function of guiding infants through a transitional stage. Shrines and sanctuaries were built to Eileithyia in caves, another symbol associated with birthing and the passage from fertile darkness into the light of the world. Dogs and horses are the animals associated with her.

Eileithyia is seen as a sacred nursemaid as well as a midwife. There are several figures depicted in Hellenic art who are referred to as Eileithyiai, suggesting that women who served as midwives and birth attendants were called by the goddess's name. Artemis is referred to as an Eileithyiai, in her guise of aide to laboring women.

Hathor

Referred to as the Great Mother Cow of Egypt, Hathor was a goddess who predated Isis, and some of her attributes were absorbed by the later goddess.

Hathor, like Eileithyia, became known as a kind of birth attendant. Some Egyptian texts speak of the Seven (or Nine) Hathors who attend the births of kings or gods, serving as oracles regarding the child's future and fate. Hathor's protection was invoked for the safety and protection of pregnant women and children. Interestingly enough, the priestesses (and priests) of Hathor were oracles as well as midwives, and as such they would interpret dreams for people who brought questions to their temples. The association between the divinatory nature of dreams and the nature of childbirth is a common one: There is a natural desire to know the future of a new life. There is also the commonly held belief that the birth of a child opens a portal between the worlds through which observations of a divinatory nature may be obtained.

Hathor is often portrayed as a woman with a cow's ears or a cow's head. She is depicted wearing the curved horn headdress that Isis later adopted. Her symbols are the sistrum and the mirror, and the animal she is associated with is, of course, the cow.

Haumea

The Polynesian goddess of fertility, labor, and childbirth, Haumea is said to be the mother of Pele, the famous volcano goddess of the Hawaiian Islands.

Some myths tell that Haumea took human form and called herself La'ila'i, while others correlate her with the goddess Papa, ancestress of the Hawaiian people.

Haumea's myths also speak of her changing her age and returning to marry her descendants to further the family line and increase the population. Children were born from several parts of her body, not only her womb, pointing to her tremendous fertility and power as a creatrix (or creatress). Her association with this fertility connects her to all living things, not only human women.

She is associated with abundance of food, possessing a stick called Makalei that can summon fish, and a tree of infinite fruit and leaves (in some myths she becomes the breadfruit tree itself, or hides her current husband within it).

The etymology of Haumea's name suggests that it is connected to *hanamea*, or "sacred birth."

Hecate

A Greek and Roman goddess of Thracian origin, Hecate is a goddess of liminal stages, transformations, and change. To see a goddess like Hecate listed among goddesses associated with birth may be a bit of a surprise to those who know her as a goddess of the underworld, revenge, or witchcraft, but one of Hecate's epithets is Divine Midwife. As a goddess of the crossroads, Hecate is associated with transition. In Greek myth, Hecate is one of the midwives attending Gaea, and it is

Hecate who hides the infant Zeus to protect him from Cronus, who has eaten each of the preceding infants Gaea has delivered.

As a liminal goddess, Hecate is a protecting figure for the pregnant woman, standing at the place of transition from one state to another. Liminal points were thought to be dangerous, for doorways through which an individual passes from one state to another were perceived as weak points through which evil spirits could also intrude. Another of her epithets is Kourotrophos, Nurse of the Children and Protectress of Mankind. In iconology she is often portrayed with a knife, which is said to be used to sever the umbilical cord. Early depictions also show her with a torch, lighting the path from the darkness of the earth and womb to the light above. In the Greek pantheon, Hecate is also perceived as a goddess of the earth and of fertility.

Heket

The Egyptian goddess of midwifery, Heket (variously spelled as Heqet and Heget) is portrayed as a frog or a frog-headed woman. She is associated with the last stages of pregnancy as well as childbirth itself. Midwives took her as their patroness, and indeed her priestesses trained as midwives. The frog was respected as a symbol of fertility in Egypt, for the annual spawning of millions of frogs that took place after the flooding of the Nile provided them with an excellent environment for reproduction.

Ix Chel

Ix Chel is the Mayan snake goddess of pregnancy and labor, earth and the moon, and weavers. She is said to nurse women through nights of labor.

Ix Chel is also associated with the rainbow, likely due to her love for the sun god and her own association with water and rain. Ix Chel also sent rains to nourish the crops, thus she is also associated with fertility of harvest, and the resulting produce. Ix Chel carries a jar that, when overturned, allows the fertile waters to flow. These waters may be seen not only as rains and floods, but as the waters of creation and the stuff of life itself as well. As a weaver, Ix Chel is also seen as having the power to create life and fortune through weaving. Shaman and anthropologist Barbara Tedlock says:

> For millennia, women the world over have sat together spinning, knotting, weaving, and sewing. These rhythmic acts of unraveling and tying together can be seen as expressions of unity and hope in the face of the reality of change, destruction, and death....Women's rituals surrounding the weaving of cloth often evoke those performed during childbirth, and the feminine shamanic path addresses both activities, as it equates spinning, knotting, and weaving a textile with the development and birth of a fetus. It's important to realize that the very processes of spinning and weaving, like those of birth, call for the ability to access the spirit world for the power to create something new.

Thus, the practical preparation for a new baby expressed in knitting and sewing new clothes and bedding also has a spiritual aspect to it.

Both snakes and dragonflies are associated with Ix Chel. The serpent is another common symbol found associated with goddesses of childbirth. The snake is a chthonic image, meaning it's associated with the underworld, and thus the serpent is also associated with earth. The dragonfly is a symbol of transformation, drawn from its metamorphosis from nymph to dragonfly, and of joy, clarity, and piercing through illusion. The dragonfly sang over Ix Chel's body when her father had struck her down for loving the Sun, bringing about a rebirth and a second life for the goddess.

Ix Chel is associated with women's cycles, both the cycle of fertility and reproduction and the overarching transition from Maiden through Crone. This is a common association with a goddess connected to crops and the moon.

Kuan Yin

An East Asian goddess of compassion revered in Korea, Japan, Vietnam, and China, Kuan Yin's patronage extends over women and children because of her association with compassion, mercy, and love. Laboring women can invoke her to help with pain and problems encountered in childbirth; women attempting to conceive can invoke her in the form of a fertility figure. She is seen as a protecting figure for all those in trouble and danger, and so quite naturally emerges as a figure associated with childbirth.

As Kuan Yin is also a bodhisattva, a figure who aids others in achieving enlightenment, she can be invoked for insight and illumination, and can help you understand the spiritual aspects of your pregnancy.

The willow is sacred to Kuan Yin, as are jasmine, lily, water lily, and lotus. Pearls and jade are the stones associated with her, while carp, dolphins, and dragons are the creatures linked to her.

Lucina

The Roman goddess of easing pain of childbirth and protecting women in labor, *Lucina* translates as "of light," signifying the passage of child from dark womb to bright world.

Roman women who experienced difficulty conceiving would also make offerings to Lucina. Both Juno and Diana are called Lucina, which points to their associations with childbirth and women's mysteries. Like most Roman goddesses, Lucina was propitiated so that the woman could avoid difficulty in her area of power. Likewise, offerings in the form of banquets and dances were made to her after the birth of the baby as part of the cycle celebrating the new life.

Nekhebet

The vulture goddess of Ancient Egypt, Nekhebet is the patroness of women in labor. She may be equated with the Greek Eileithyia. Nekhebet is depicted in art as a woman with a vulture headdress, or as a woman with a vulture's head.

In Egyptian myth, Nekhebet attended the births of gods and kings. Like many other goddesses associated with childbirth, she is also associated with the moon and sometimes the sun. In her role of guardian of the newly born infant pharaoh, she was referred to as the Great White Cow of Nekheb, again underscoring the reverence with which many cultures held the cow in terms of childbirth.

Nephthys

Nephthys is more commonly seen as a shadow goddess, a shadow companion to the popular Isis. Nonetheless, she is included in certain myths as a birth attendant, and this suggests that despite her darker nature, Nephthys performs an important function during the rite of passage known as childbirth. The transitional state of the rite suggests that the laboring woman has connections to more than one realm, which means that she can see and comprehend the importance of death in this act that confirms life. The two concepts of life and death are very close during childbirth. Additionally, the darker nature of Nephthys may also be represented by the darkness of the womb, and the brighter nature represented by the light of the sun or moon into which the child is born. The passage from one state to another is made ceremonious by the presence of Nephthys and Isis, representations of the two extremes.

Sometimes Nephthys is portrayed with vulture wings. Vultures are associated with death and decay, but also with motherhood, for vultures are said to travel in mother-child pairs. Thus Nephthys represents both the life and death energies that childbirth encompasses.

Chapter 4

Using Energy for Strength, Support, and Insight

Pregnancy is one long liminal stage, a transformation that yields a shift into a new role. It's important to have access to a variety of aids to support yourself spiritually throughout the journey. This chapter focuses on correspondences and energies you can use throughout your pregnancy for strength, support, and insight.

Working with the Elements

When pregnant, you may feel out of sync with your environment due to all the changes and transformations going on in your body. How can you relate to the world around you when you feel out of touch with your own physical self?

Apart from working with a goddess, the most basic way to keep in touch with the shifts and transitions occurring in your body and personal energy is by working with the four physical elements. These four elements—earth, air, fire, and water—are the building blocks of the physical world. They are also cornerstones of most neo-pagan practice, symbolizing a variety of concepts and associated energies.

By working with the elements one on one, you can explore your connection to those basic building blocks as well as how they manifest within you. With a better understanding of how those elements interact with your own energy while you are pregnant, you can gain a clearer view of the changes occurring in your emotional and spiritual selves, as well as your physical body.

The meditations included here are deliberately similar, in order for you to better see the differences and sense the shifts in energy while you perform them. Do them more than once throughout your pregnancy, whenever you feel the need to do one or all four, to help rebalance your energy. For each element, two meditations are given; experiment with both options, or choose whichever one speaks to you at the time.

Earth

The element of earth is a wonderful element to work with while pregnant. On the most basic level, it is a stable, grounding element, and thus is something upon which you can call to help ground and relax you when you're tense, stressed, wobbly, or in any other undesired state.

Earth is also the element associated with fertility and abundance. The earth is what nourishes and grows all green living things. The term *fruition* derives from the completion of the life cycle from seed to fruit; and the term *fertile* describes the active state of something ready and able to reproduce. The element of earth is traditionally perceived as having a feminine energy and it is traditionally associated with the physical body.

- ❖ Many of the mother goddesses are associated with earth, such as Demeter, Gaea, Rhea, and Cybele.
- ❖ Tools associated with earth include disks, plates, stones, crystals, sand, earth, pebbles, and shields.
- ❖ Animals associated with earth include cattle, bison and buffalo, oxen, bears, wolves, dogs, and deer.

EARTH MEDITATION

YOU WILL NEED

- ❖ Your journal and a writing tool (see Chapter 6 for information about creating a spiritual pregnancy journal; otherwise, use your regular Book of Shadows, magical journal, or diary)
- ❖ A towel or blanket

DIRECTIONS

1. Prepare your space as per your usual meditation procedure. If you are not accustomed to meditation, see the basic outline in Chapter 5. Have your spiritual pregnancy journal on hand with a pen or pencil.

2. While lying down to meditate is not usually recommended, it's required for this meditation. Lie down on a towel or a blanket, or on a rug. Center and ground.

3. Close your eyes and breathe calmly and regularly. As you exhale, allow your body to relax. With every exhalation, feel heavier and heavier.

4. Visualize yourself lying in a grassy field. Imagine yourself sinking into the ground, becoming one with it.

5. Sense the energy of the earth around you. Allow it to merge with your own energy. Be earth.

6. Stay like this for as long as you desire. When you are ready to end the meditation, imagine rising to the surface of the earth again. Feel the change in the air, and in the sense of the energy.

7. Visualize yourself back in your physical location. Center and ground again. Take three deep breaths, then open your eyes.

8. Stretch carefully and sit up. In your spiritual pregnancy journal, write about your meditation experience and the things you felt.

ALTERNATE EARTH MEDITATION

For this meditation, you will need to wear old clothes or clothes you don't mind getting dirty. Make sure to wear a separate top and bottom.

YOU WILL NEED

❖ A large towel
❖ A bowl of rich earth (do not use sand or salt)
❖ Your journal and a writing tool

DIRECTIONS

1. Spread the towel on the ground. If it's not long enough for you to lie flat on, spread the towel crosswise so that it will be under your abdomen, stretching out to the sides.

2. If you are concerned about the energy associated with the earth, you may purify it before you use it. Hold your hands above the bowl of earth and visualize white, silver, or golden light pouring from your hands into the earth. Visualize any negative energy buried within the earth dissolving away as the light hits it.

3. Lie down on the towel, with the bowl of earth by your side and within reach of your hand. Center and ground. Then pull up your shirt so that your abdomen is exposed. If you need to, fold down the waistband of your pants as well.

4. Close your eyes and breathe calmly and regularly. Release tension with each exhalation, and allow your body to relax and feel heavier with each breath.

5. When you are ready, lift your hand and touch the earth in the bowl. Burrow your fingers into it, allowing the grains of earth to roll over them. Note how the earth feels to your fingers, then sense the energy of the earth.

6. When you are ready, gently scoop up some of the earth in your hand. Bring it over your abdomen, and gently allow some earth to trickle down onto your skin. If your abdomen is too sensitive for this, lower your hand and gently place the earth onto your belly. Note how it feels, both physically and spiritually. Place more earth on your abdomen. Run your fingers through it carefully, moving it around. Spread it out, or draw designs in it. As you do, draw the energy of the earth directly into your abdomen.

7. When you feel ready, gently brush off the earth from your abdomen onto the towel below you. Take three deep breaths, center and ground again, and open your eyes. Stretch carefully and sit up. Write down your impressions and experiences in your spiritual pregnancy journal.

Water

Water is considered the element of transformation. It is traditionally seen to possess feminine energy. Water is an element that is patient but deep. If overlooked or undervalued, it can command attention by presenting with a tsunami or a flood. Think of the power contained within a waterfall.

Water is also associated with emotions. If you're seeking to balance your emotions because you're feeling overwhelmed by the sudden shifts in mood, or if you are uncomfortable with the extremes to which your emotions seem to be tending, work with the element of water to try to understand your emotions and rebalance them. Water is an excellent element to work with during pregnancy, as it is the basis of your blood, which increases by 40 to 50 percent during your pregnancy to meet the metabolic needs of both your body and that of your child. The chemicals and hormones in your body are distributed by water, and the amniotic fluid surrounding the fetus is also formed mostly of water.

Water can be calm, as in ponds or small streams, or strong and relentless like the currents in large deep rivers and ocean tides. Tides are another excellent example of how the element of water manifests in pregnancy: What flows in, flows out. Everything in your pregnancy is part of a cycle. Your emotions aren't random, as they sometimes appear to be; they respond to fluctuations in your chemical makeup, which in turn responds to diet, the needs of the fetus, and the readjustments your body makes as required throughout the pregnancy.

❖ Mother goddesses associated with water include Isis and Brigid.

❖ Tools associated with water are cauldrons, chalices and cups, seashells, bowls, and sea salt.

❖ Animals associated with water include fish, dolphin, whales, waterfowl and sea birds, frogs, turtles, seals, crabs, and otters.

WATER MEDITATION

YOU WILL NEED

❖ Your journal and a writing tool

❖ A towel or blanket

DIRECTIONS

1. Prepare your space as per your usual meditation procedure. If you are not accustomed to meditation, see the basic outline in Chapter 5. Have your spiritual pregnancy journal on hand with a pen or pencil.

2. Lie down on a towel or a blanket, or on a rug; or, if you prefer, sit in a chair. Center and ground.

3. Close your eyes and breathe calmly and regularly. As you exhale, allow your body to relax. With every exhalation, feel yourself relaxing more and more.

4. Visualize your surroundings slowly changing to a warm and safe body of water. Feel the flow of water below and around you. Feel the movement of the waves and the surface gently cradling you and dipping you soothingly up and down. Sense the energy of the water as it flows around and beneath you. Then allow the energy of the water to merge with your own energy. Feel the calming, cleansing energy of water; allow it to purify your fears and doubts.

5. Stay like this for as long as you desire. When you are ready to end the meditation, imagine the water cradling you slowly fading, to be replaced by your physical environment once again. Center and ground again. Take three deep breaths, then open your eyes.

6. Stretch carefully and sit up. In your spiritual pregnancy journal, write about your experience and the things you felt.

ALTERNATE WATER MEDITATION

For this meditation, you will need to wear old clothes or clothes you don't mind getting wet. Make sure to wear a separate top and bottom.

YOU WILL NEED

❖ A large towel
❖ A bowl of water
❖ A small hand towel
❖ Your journal and a writing tool

DIRECTIONS

1. Spread the towel on the ground. If it's not long enough for you to lie flat on, spread the towel crosswise so that it will be under your abdomen, stretching out to the sides.

2. If you are concerned about the energy associated with the water, you may purify and consecrate it before you use it. Add a pinch of salt and stir the water three times counterclockwise, visualizing the negative energy contained within it evaporating.

3. Lie down on the towel, with the bowl of water by your side and within reach of your hand. Have the smaller hand towel within reach as well. Center and ground. Then pull up your shirt so that your abdomen is exposed. If you need to, fold down the waistband of your pants as well.

4. Close your eyes and breathe calmly and regularly. Release tension with each exhalation, and allow your body to relax and feel heavier with each breath.

5. When you are ready, lift your hand and touch the water in the bowl. Gently swish your fingers in it. Note how the water feels to your fingers, then sense the energy of the water.

6. When you are ready, gently scoop up some of the water in your hand. Bring it over your abdomen and allow it to trickle down onto your skin, or bring your hand directly to your belly and gently rub the water over your skin. Note how it feels, both physically and spiritually. Place more water on your abdomen, and play with it. As you do, draw the energy of the water directly into your abdomen.

7. When you feel ready, take the hand towel and gently dry your abdomen. Take three deep breaths, center and ground again, and open your eyes. Stretch carefully and sit up. Write about your impressions and experiences in your spiritual pregnancy journal.

Air

Air is associated with movement, thought, perception, and knowledge. It is traditionally perceived as having masculine energy. Air is also the element that governs breathing. Give your body the gifts of breathing well and ensuring you have good posture during your pregnancy. These gifts will provide more oxygen for your blood, which in turn will nourish your own body and oxygenate your fetus. Interestingly enough, the higher levels of progesterone during pregnancy cause you to take deeper breaths while pregnant. Correct breathing is especially important during later pregnancy, when the uterus presses against the diaphragm and may cause shortness of breath. All in all, you may become very aware of your breath during your pregnancy, as your physical activity and position affect it.

Breathing is also a technique for coping with the physical demands of labor. When you attend to the rhythm of breathing, either in a natural or a structured pattern, your mind can simultaneously focus on something other than the physical stress and provide relaxation.

- ❖ Mother goddesses associated with air are Arianrhod and Isis.
- ❖ Tools associated with air are wands, feathers, fans, chimes, ribbons, flags, incense, potpourri, flowers, and spears.
- ❖ Animals associated with air include birds and insects (especially the dragonfly and butterfly).

AIR MEDITATION

Do this meditation outside if possible.

YOU WILL NEED

❖ Your journal and a writing tool
❖ A blanket or towel

DIRECTIONS

1. Prepare your space as per your usual meditation procedure. If you are not accustomed to meditation, see the basic outline in Chapter 5. Have your spiritual pregnancy journal on hand with a pen or pencil.

2. Lie down on a towel or a blanket, or sit on the ground or in a chair. Center and ground.

3. Close your eyes and breathe calmly and regularly. As you exhale, allow your body to relax. With every exhalation, feel more tension leave your body until you are fully relaxed.

4. Open yourself to the feel of the air around you. Notice how it moves, how it flows, how it changes direction. Listen to how it moves tree leaves and grass. Visualize yourself being fully surrounded by air. Sense the energy of the air around you. Consciously draw the energy into your body as you inhale. Allow it to merge with your own energy. Be air.

5. Stay like this for as long as you desire. When you are ready to end the meditation, visualize yourself back in your physical location. Feel the chair or the ground beneath you. Center and ground again. Take three deep breaths, then open your eyes.

6. Stretch carefully and sit up. In your spiritual pregnancy journal, write about your experience and the things you felt.

ALTERNATE AIR MEDITATION

For this meditation, make sure to wear a separate top and bottom. It should be performed outside.

YOU WILL NEED

❖ A blanket or towel
❖ Your journal and a writing tool

DIRECTIONS

1. Spread the blanket on the ground and lie down on it. Center and ground. Close your eyes and breathe calmly and regularly. Release tension with each exhalation, and allow your body to relax and feel heavier with each breath.

2. When you are ready, lift up your shirt to expose your abdomen (you may wish to fold down the waistband of your pants as well). Feel the air moving over your skin. Note how the air feels physically, then sense the energy of the air.

3. Stay this way as long as feels comfortable, and when you feel ready, slowly pull down your shirt to cover your abdomen again. Take three deep breaths, center and ground again, and open your eyes.

4. Stretch carefully and sit up. Write about your impressions and experiences in your spiritual pregnancy journal.

5. If inclement weather keeps you inside, do this meditation by gently fanning your abdomen with a hand fan instead.

Fire

Fire is the element associated with passion and creativity. Gestation is the living embodiment of creativity, the act of forming and nurturing a new life into being. Even if you sit calmly with your eyes closed, your body is still hard at work creating, nourishing, and growing.

Fire is also often perceived to be the very spark of life that animates the spirit, and sometimes as evidence of Divinity itself. Fire is a sacred thing in several cultures. The sun is the most accessible symbol associated with the element of fire. Fire is considered to be a masculine element.

❖ Mother goddesses associated with fire include Brigid.
❖ Tools associated with fire include candles, matches, charcoal, and blades such as knives, swords, and axes.
❖ Creatures associated with fire include lions, dragons, salamanders, and snakes.

FIRE MEDITATION

YOU WILL NEED
❖ Your journal and a writing tool

DIRECTIONS

1. Prepare your space as per your usual meditation procedure. If you are not accustomed to meditation, see the basic outline in Chapter 5. Have your spiritual pregnancy journal on hand with a pen or pencil.

2. Sit comfortably in a chair. Center and ground. Close your eyes and breathe calmly and regularly. As you exhale, allow your body to relax. With every exhalation, feel yourself relaxing more and more.

3. Visualize a patch of flames forming in front of you. Feel the warmth and the life contained within them. Slowly visualize yourself stepping forward until you are within the flames and they surround you completely. They do not burn; rather, they energize. Feel the flicker of warm and safe flames, and sense

the energy of the fire around you. Allow the energy of the fire to merge with your own energy.

4. Stay like this for as long as you desire. Open yourself to the energy of fire; let it fill you and acquaint you with the true nature of fire. Feel yourself invigorated, impassioned, and very alive. When you are ready to end the meditation, imagine the flames around you slowly fading. Center and ground again. Take three deep breaths, then open your eyes.

5. Stretch carefully and sit up. In your spiritual pregnancy journal, write about your experience and the things you felt and observed.

ALTERNATE FIRE MEDITATION

For this meditation, make sure to wear a separate top and bottom. It should be performed outside on a sunny day.

YOU WILL NEED

❖ A towel or blanket
❖ Your journal and a writing tool

DIRECTIONS

1. Spread the towel or blanket on the ground and lie down on it. Close your eyes and breathe calmly and regularly. Release tension with each exhalation, and allow your body to relax and feel heavier with each breath.

2. When you are ready, lift up your shirt to expose your abdomen (you may wish to fold down the waistband of your pants as well). Feel the warmth of the sun on your skin. Note how the sun feels physically, then sense the energy of the sunlight. Allow the energy of the sun to soak into your abdomen.

3. Stay this way as long as feels comfortable, and when you feel ready, slowly pull your shirt back down over your abdomen. Take three deep breaths, center and ground, and open your eyes. Stretch carefully and sit up. Write about your impressions and experiences in your spiritual pregnancy journal.

4. If inclement weather keeps you inside, do this meditation by exposing your abdomen to candlelight or firelight instead. Make sure to secure candles in proper holders on a steady surface, and far enough away that there is no chance of accidentally hitting them as you move. If you choose to light a fire in a fireplace for this exercise, have a secure fire screen set in front of it before you begin your meditation. In both instances, be certain to have a fire extinguisher or bucket of sand handy in case of an accident.

The Tarot

One of the tools commonly found in the neo-pagan's possession is a deck of tarot cards. Traditionally used for divination, the tarot deck also offers you a rich meditation tool. Whether you work with tarot on a regular basis or not, meditating on certain cards can provide you with insight into pregnancy-related concepts and issues. If you do not own a tarot deck, you can find many beautiful illustrations of the cards online.

Here are three ways you can use a tarot card as a meditative tool:

1. Use a particular tarot card as a visual focus (good pregnancy-related choices are described later in this section). Gaze at the

card and allow associations to arise in your mind. Record these in your journal when you are done.

2. Imagine walking into the image depicted on the card. Explore the environment. Be open to messages and observations inspired by what you see. If the card portrays a specific individual, she or he (or it) may initiate speech with you; learn from them. Or other individuals may appear in the landscape and converse with you.

3. Imagine meeting the person portrayed on the card and speaking with him or her.

The following four tarot cards are drawn from the Major Arcana. The Major Arcana tends to be more richly detailed than the Minor Arcana, which is often illustrated only with "pips," or the number of items representing a given suit. Each of these Major Arcana cards has certain themes and associations that make it a good focus for pregnancy-related meditation.

❖ **THE HIGH PRIESTESS:** This card represents instinctual knowledge and often carries the message, "Trust yourself." The High Priestess also represents wisdom, intuition, and secret knowledge. These are all things you draw upon throughout your pregnancy, both consciously and unconsciously; secret knowledge is also uncovered as you progress through the sacred mystery. You can read books on pregnancy until the cows come home, but until you begin going through the pregnancy itself, you can't internalize the information; it won't mean as much. If you are looking for a card to use as a focus for attuning to the mysteries of motherhood while pregnant, The High Priestess is the one.

❖ **THE EMPRESS:** This card represents the creatrix aspect of the Goddess, the great womb in which things gestate and form. Whereas The High Priestess helps you connect to the instinctual knowledge that will help you do something, The Empress gives you the physical means through which to bring it forth. The Empress card is strongly associated with mothers, and it symbolizes the qualities of motherhood such as patience, generosity, love, and nurturing. This is an excellent card to work with if you are seeking to treat fertility problems.

❖ **THE STAR:** This card represents hope, the future, spiritual insight, inspiration, and potential. It is a card to turn to for help and support throughout your journey. The Star card can also be valuable when you feel uncertain about the future, or uneasy about your pregnancy in any respect.

❖ **THE SUN:** This card is traditionally associated with children, pleasure, success, and joy. The Sun is an excellent card upon which to meditate when you want to look ahead and focus on the successful completion of your pregnancy. Sometimes you may get bogged down in the day-to-day toil of pregnancy and have difficulty seeing beyond the discomfort or the seemingly unending months, particularly when the pregnancy is in its third trimester. Meditating on The Sun card helps remind you that your toil is a loving work, honoring both the Goddess and yourself, and also your child, the literal fruit of your labor.

Working with Animal Energy

Like the tarot, working with animal energies is a common neo-pagan practice. Animals are frequently used as symbols in ritual and spellwork, and as teachers or guides on a spiritual level. People frequently refer to a certain animal as being a totem for them. In neo-pagan parlance, this is an animal that symbolizes an aspect of you or an animal chosen as a helper to reflect certain positive qualities in yourself, or qualities you wish to cultivate. In correct use of the word, however, a totem is the permanent protector or patron of a specific group of people found within a shamanic culture.

In more specific terms, what many neo-pagans term a *personal totem* is more correctly an *animal spirit guide*, a teacherlike animal spirit who offers you wisdom, guidance, and energy. These guides can be linked to you for a limited time period, meaning that the guide will move on when you have accomplished what you or it needed to do, or for a longer period of time, functioning as a companion or guardian whose energy and associations you can learn from or attune to. These animal spirit guides can be specifically called or invoked by you through ritual and linked to you if they acquiesce, or they may present themselves to you without forewarning or preparation on your part with a message or a lesson to impart.

If you are interested in working with a specific animal energy while you are pregnant, here is a sequence of simple methods through which you may get to know the animal, its energy, and its areas of strength and power:

1. Research the animal. Read up on its mythological associations, habitats, diet, mating behavior, life cycle, and so forth. Learn as much as you can about both the physical attributes and the spiritual attributes.

2. Meditate on the actual animal itself. Use a picture of the animal as a visual focus.

3. Meditate on the attributes and associations of the animal.

4. Visualize the animal in your mind, and embrace whatever associations come to mind: ideas, thoughts, sounds, scents, words, and so forth. Write these down in your spiritual journal.

5. Create a shrine to the animal, or include an image of the animal on your pregnancy shrine.

6. Honor the animal spirit by giving it a suitable offering, according to its associations and/or diet.

7. Create a representation of the animal in the form of a drawing, sculpture, poem, or story. Place it on your pregnancy shrine or altar, or offer it to nature by burning it and scattering the ashes with reverence, burying it, or releasing it into a moving body of water.

Many animals have been associated with pregnancy throughout history. The following sections describe some totems and their spirit energies as they have been symbolically related to fertility, pregnancy, and childbirth.

Rabbit and Hare

The rabbit is almost always perceived as a fertility symbol in Western culture. On a very basic level, this derives from its ubiquitous presence and its legendary reproductive cycle. The turbo-charged reproductive cycle of the rabbit exists for a very plain purpose: The rabbit is one of nature's basic prey animals; it serves as food for a myriad of predators. This basic purpose aside, the rabbit is an excellent animal with which to work while pregnant. The rabbit is also associated with the Goddess and with the Otherworld as symbolized by the underground. The association with the underground also connects the rabbit to the element of earth, an element associated with stability, fertility, and abundance. The rabbit is also associated with the quality of liminality—the state of being on the verge of something—and the related concept of transition. The rabbit is often seen at dusk and at dawn, two liminal times, and in environments that possess liminal geography such as the borders of woods and meadows. These qualities are valuable for the pregnant woman, who is herself in a liminal state, transitioning between pre-pregnancy and post-pregnancy. The connection to the Otherworld offers you the opportunity for insight into the cycle of life at the point between death and rebirth, where many European cultures situate the soul's rejuvenation and preparation for a new life. Some cultures place unborn children in this luminous Otherworld as they prepare to be born. In dreams and meditations, you can reach out to this Otherworld and send messages of love and welcome to your child, whoever he or she may be.

The rabbit is very sensitive. It is strongly connected to its environment and in touch with its surroundings, mainly because it is constantly on the lookout for predators. You can use this quality to be in touch with your environment, too, to sense when you should ground, when you should find a calmer place to be, and when to relax your shields in order to absorb as much of the comforting energy around you as possible. Being in touch with your environment means that you can act to protect yourself and your child before there is a full-blown problem or threat, or act to take advantage of any positive energy present to build up your reserves or give yourself a bit of a break.

Specifically, the rabbit is associated with Hecate. It is also often associated with Eostre, a minor goddess of Eastern European origin who personifies the season of spring and new beginnings.

The hare, an animal often mislabeled as a rabbit, can conceive while pregnant. The hare is associated with fertility, the moon, and new life. It is strongly associated with physical transformation, which makes it an ideal totem with which to work during pregnancy. The hare tends to be associated with wisdom more than the rabbit. It is also a trickster figure, carrying messages from the gods but also misleading humankind. Hares do not burrow; rather, they birth and rest in bowl-like depressions on the earth's surface. Young hares are born fully furred and with their eyes open, and they learn to function as adults quickly, probably due to the lack of defense that their physical home offers them. In ancient Greek culture, a hare's genitals would sometimes be carried to avert barrenness. Hares are associated with Freyja, the Teutonic goddess of love, sexuality, and women's mysteries; Artemis, the Greek goddess of wilderness creatures and the hunt; and Aphrodite, the Greek goddess of love and beauty.

Swan

The swan is a thing of grace and beauty, two concepts that women in the modern Western world often have difficulty recognizing in themselves while pregnant. Stereotypes and cultural emphasis on thin willowy bodies create a difficult context within which pregnant women must struggle in order to perceive themselves as beautiful. Working with swan energy can help balance the negative physical self-image that arises during pregnancy. If you find yourself out of step with your body as your center of gravity shifts and your physical dimensions seem to change every day, align yourself with the swan to help regain a sense of control and grace.

The swan is associated with the elements of water and air. The water association links it to dreams and the realm of emotion, as well as transformation. The air association links it to thought and knowledge, more logic-based realms. In short, the swan offers the potential for balance between head and heart, a balance that is sometimes difficult to maintain during pregnancy. This balance may be symbolized by the swan's main identifying feature, the long and supple neck that connects the head with the body, representing the flexible connection between head and heart.

The swan is also associated with dreams, which may be perceived as a method by which your mind communicates with the Otherworld, the realm of spirit. The swan can be invoked as an aid in contacting your child as it grows, allowing you to reassure them and communicate your love for them.

The swan is very protective both of the nesting mother and of cygnets once they have hatched, and for this reason is often perceived as being associated with parenthood as well. White is the color of the majority of swan species, which links it with innocence and purity, and thus its association is extended to children in general as well.

Specifically, the swan is associated with the swan maiden Caer Ibormeith, an Irish goddess of prophecy and sleep who is part of the

"Dream of Aengus" myth. Caer transformed into a swan at Samhain and remained a swan for a year, transforming into a human again the following Samhain for the next year. She appeared to Aengus, the god of youth and beauty, in a dream. Wasting away from lovesickness, Aengus searched for Caer and finally discovered her at a lake full of swans. He correctly identified her in her swan form among the others and transformed into a swan himself, and they flew away together, singing beautiful music.

Using the swan to help you communicate with your unborn child through dreams and meditations can help you gain a sense of comfort with your pregnancy and lessen your sense of being someone to whom something is happening, as opposed to a full participant. For a ritual that uses the swan as a symbol and guide to help you communicate with your child, see later on in this chapter.

Elephant

The elephant bears the honor of being the mammal with the longest gestational period, at twenty-two months. The weight of an average elephant calf is approximately 225 pounds! The elephant is an excellent animal to call upon to reinforce your patience during pregnancy. If nothing else, the elephant can serve as inspiration for gratitude among human women for the fact that our young gestate for only nine calendar months and are born at an average weight of about 7.5 pounds.

The elephant is a symbol of fertility in India, as well as a symbol of royalty. Both these associations are important for the pregnant woman, for she is living proof of fertility, as well as being a queen among women for carrying life within her. In so doing, she is sacred. Elephants also represent power and strength.

Elephants live in communities separated by sex. Cows and calves live together, and an older, experienced cow leads this herd. This leader may be viewed as a crone matriarch figure. The female community is consequently made up of child, mother, and crone, providing a complete and balanced representation of the three aspects associated with the Goddess. The elephant is thus associated with family and society, social environments in which individuals care for one another and draw strength from others in the community. Males usually live on the fringes of a herd or in loose informal bachelor herds.

Elephants raise their young in a community atmosphere. Unlike many other mammals, elephants are not born with a full set of survival skills. The older females in the community teach life skills to calves. In addition to this, a mother elephant will be aided by selected females of the herd to serve as aunts or godmothers to the new calf, assisting it physically as the herd travels, and guarding and guiding it as it grows, allowing the mother to feed herself and produce as much milk as possible and to maximize the quality of her milk.

The elephant is associated with the element of earth, which further supports its connections to strength, fertility, and patience. It is associated with Ganesha, the elephant-headed Hindu god of success, wealth and abundance, fidelity, intelligence, and wisdom; and with Malini, an elephant-headed goddess of the river of the same name. Malini is associated with protection from bad fortune and accidents. (Interestingly enough, one of Ganesha's origin myths has him being formed of turmeric by his mother Parvati, who then breathes life into him: another example of a goddess creating life with no input from a male partner. An alternate origin story has Parvati's bathwater being poured into the river, and Malini then birthing Ganesha.)

The elephant is an excellent totem for pregnant women to work with. Patience, strength, supportive family and community, power, and fertility are all associations that offer guidance.

Stork

The stork is a traditional symbol associated with birth in Western culture. It is also linked with Juno, the Roman goddess of home, children, and family loyalty. Folk wisdom has it that a stork nesting on your roof will bring good fortune to the household. Storks have been widely associated with parenting and family throughout the Western world, likely attributed to the behavior of a mated pair in and around their nest. The earliest recorded mention of storks delivering children is found in Dutch and German folktales.

The stork is a shorebird, and thus is associated with water and earth, as well as air. Like the swan, it represents a balance between emotions and logical thought. Also like the swan, it is a caring and dedicated parent to its young.

Storks lack a syrinx (a bird's vocal cords) and are therefore mute. The lack of a physical voice suggests the importance of wordless communication, perhaps in the form of internal communication, rather than talking in a logical dialogue. The stork is thus an ideal totem with which to work if you seek to facilitate or strengthen your communication with your unborn child. The stork uses physical movement to communicate, utilizing both body language and the clacking of its beak. This suggests the importance of communicating with your own body throughout your pregnancy, as well as communicating with your child. Be sensitive to your own body's needs and desires, and respond to them thoughtfully and with love.

Cow

The cow is an almost universal symbol of fertility and motherhood. In several cultures, cattle have been associated with wealth, prosperity, and abundance, and they were one of the earliest forms of currency. Cattle provide humankind with food, both meat and dairy, and also with power for hauling and mechanical purposes.

In Hindu society, the cow is sacred. The flesh of cattle is not consumed: The animals are honored and kept only for dairy and work. According to Hindu religion, the cow brings humankind five gifts: milk, curds, butter, urine (used to medicate), and manure (dried and used as fuel), as well as calves, who serve to perpetuate the gifts. In several cultures, the cow is thought to have been a cosmic mother, birthing and nursing the world. In Norse mythology, a cow not only nourished the primordial hermaphroditic giant Ymir with her milk but also licked the ice of the frozen world, melting it and releasing the first god, Buri.

In Egypt, there existed a mythology text called *The Book of the Heavenly Cow*, which appears in a handful of pharaonic tombs, telling the story of man's rebellion against the sun god and the subsequent introduction of death to the human race. The Heavenly Cow is the goddess Nut (or Nuet, or Nuit), who is the sky goddess arching over the earth to protect it from the darkness and demons beyond. She is also the mother of the gods Osiris, Isis, Set, and Nephthys, four of the most recognizable Egyptian deities.

The cow is associated with the goddesses Hera and Hathor. Brigid, in her Catholic cognate Saint Bridget (often called Saint Brigid), is sometimes portrayed with milk pails, and one of her epithets is Brigid of the Kine, a term indicating a collection of cattle. The Hindu goddess Parvati rides a white cow.

Other Animal Totems

There's nothing stopping you from working with other energies during your pregnancy. If you are drawn to work with the energy of an animal not mentioned here, by all means do so. Meditate, read as much as you can on the animal, and try to discover what lesson the animal spirit has for you at this time. Also research how your regular animal guides handle pregnancy and parenting; there may be something important for you to learn from them as well.

Swan Charm for Attuning to Your Unborn Child

This spell creates a small charm or fetish for you to use to help strengthen your connection to your unborn child. The spell calls for Fimo or some other craft polymer clay that requires baking, but you can use regular self-hardening clay or homemade salt dough if you prefer. Follow the baking directions for your clay of choice.

This spell creates a small, compact swan figure to avoid potential cracking and breakage. If this spell appeals to you and you wish to make a larger figurine, use a wire framework for the neck and head and extend the wire into the body to provide as much support as possible.

YOU WILL NEED

- ❖ 1 teaspoon jasmine herb
- ❖ Mortar and pestle
- ❖ Approximately 1 ounce white Fimo (about the size of a walnut)

❖ Small moonstone (a chip is fine; make sure it's no bigger than a small marble)

❖ Needle, knife, or other tools with which to detail (optional)

❖ Foil

❖ Baking sheet

❖ Paint for the clay (optional)

❖ Copal incense

❖ Incense burner

❖ White candle

❖ Candleholder

❖ Matches or a lighter

DIRECTIONS

1. Powder the jasmine in a mortar and pestle. (If fresh, first dry it by spreading the flowers on a foil-covered baking sheet and placing them in a barely warm oven for a few minutes until crumbly to the touch.)

2. Purify and bless the jasmine, clay, and moonstone.

3. Empower the jasmine with your desire to attune to your unborn child.

4. Soften the Fimo or clay by working it with your hands. When soft enough, flatten out the Fimo with the base of your hand and sprinkle the jasmine over it. Roll up the Fimo into a ball again and knead it with your fingers until the jasmine is evenly distributed.

5. Form the Fimo into a roughly oval shape, and flatten it with the base of your hand. Press the moonstone into the center, and then fold one end of the oval up around the stone. This will be the swan's body.

6. Take the other end and draw it out slightly, using your fingers to smooth it into a cylinder shape. Bend it up and back to touch the

body and continue up to form the neck of the swan. Bend the very end forward again to form the swan's head and beak. Make sure it rests down against the neck to avoid breakage during baking or subsequent handling.

7. Adjust the shape to your liking. You may add detail with a needle or sharp knife if you like.

8. Place the swan on the foil-covered baking sheet and bake the clay as directed on the package.

9. If you so desire, you may paint the swan after it has cooled.

10. When the swan is dry and ready, bring it to your altar or pregnancy shrine. Center and ground.

11. Create sacred space or cast a circle. Light the copal incense and the white candle. Set the swan figure between the candle and incense. Say:

> *Timeless Swan,*
> *Bird of beauty and of grace,*
> *You who swim the river between this world and the world*
> *   of Spirit,*
> *Be for me a messenger.*
> *Carry my love and my hopes to my child waiting to be born.*
> *Tell my child that s/he is much loved,*
> *That s/he is welcome,*
> *And that s/he is safe.*
> *Blessed Swan,*
> *May our dreams be sweet.*
> *So may it be.*

12. Place the swan figure on your pregnancy shrine, or place it in a small bag and carry it with you in your purse or pocket. Alternatively, you may place it by your bed.

Using Stones

Stones are easy to use: The most basic way to employ them is to carry them on your person in some way, be it in a pocket or in a small bag or pouch, in order to avail yourself of their energy. Some believe that the stone itself must be touching your skin in order to lend its energy to you, and while this may not be absolutely true, it does make the energy use more direct and thus more efficient. Stones can certainly be worn on a chain as a pendant, as earrings, in rings, and set in piercing jewelry.

You can do just about anything with stones. Add them to spell bags or set them out on tables or shelves. Tuck some under your pillow or under the bed. Place them on your pregnancy shrine. Carry them loose in your purse or backpack or briefcase.

Every stone has a multitude of associations and correspondences, many of which can be applied to pregnancy, but here are the stones that are most directly associated with some aspect of pregnancy and motherhood:

❖ **MOONSTONE:** Named for the opalescent play of light that suggests the waxing and waning of the moon, this stone is associated with dreams, love, motherhood, and children. In Arab countries it is thought to bring fertility, and in India it is considered a sacred stone, capable of bringing sweet dreams. It facilitates the expression of emotion, particularly love, and for this reason can be used to help you bond with your unborn child. The moonstone is also thought to enhance intuition. It comes in a variety of soft colors such as white, pale gray, pale peach, and pale green.

❖ **MALACHITE:** A vibrant green stone with thin bands or scallops of lighter green throughout, malachite is associated with fertility, abundance, and the earth. Malachite is said to warn of impending danger. It can provide extra energy and relax physical tension, as well as calm the emotions and enhance patience. It is said to restore harmony in a physical environment. Malachite is also used to protect children and infants.

❖ **BLOODSTONE:** A dark green stone with speckles of red, the bloodstone is said to enhance courage. It is carried to promote healing in general and to protect and strengthen the blood system. It protects against miscarriage and aids the physical development of the fetus. Bloodstone is said to bestow insight regarding change.

❖ **CARNELIAN:** A red, orange, or reddish-brown stone, carnelian is strongly associated with success. It can help you make major life decisions, particularly regarding the future and your career, which can be stressful subjects during pregnancy. It enhances confidence, motivation, and creativity. Carnelian also defends against anger, sorrow, and depression, both in the carrier and those around. Carnelian is a healing stone, and it can lend energy.

The Energies of Food and Herbs

The aphorism "you are what you eat" holds particularly true during pregnancy. Many of the magical correspondences or folk wisdom benefits associated with various foods come from a visual parallel. Nuts and seeds and melons, for example, have an interior contained within a hard exterior and are often round or ovoid in shape. Certain foods are associated with pregnancy or fertility for this reason. By eating these foods you can internalize the associated energy and add it to your own.

Here are some foods associated with pregnancy:

❖ **NUTS AND SEEDS:** Because they are the reproductive fruit of a plant or tree, nuts and seeds hold great fertility energy and are frequently used for fertility magic. They are also used for wish magic, prosperity, and abundance magic.

❖ **WATERMELON:** The suggestive shape of the watermelon and other melons holds imitative energy. Additionally, it holds seeds within it, a further promise of life.

❖ **FIG:** The fig is a fruit that visually resembles the womb, and as such may be used in fertility magic.

❖ **EGG:** The egg is a common symbol of fertility. Eggs may be used in fertility magic and also as foci for safe-pregnancy spells and rituals. (See Chapter 6 for one such ritual.)

In addition, there are time-honored foods and herbs that can help ease your pregnancy discomfort. Remember, however, that too much of anything qualifies as overdosing and can harm you or your child. Following are some foods and seasonings that can be helpful to use during pregnancy:

❖ **GINGER:** Ginger makes a wonderful remedy for nausea and morning sickness. Grate fresh ginger (or slice thinly). Pour boiling water over it, then steep for about half an hour. Strain and drink a cup at a time. It can be taken hot or cold, although most people find the warm version more comforting. If you find your nausea popping up throughout the day, carry some dried or crystallized ginger with you and chew a bit when you need to. Crystallized ginger is candied, so it contains a lot of sugar; don't go overboard. (Although if you're looking for a treat, a single piece of candied ginger dipped in dark chocolate goes a long way toward making yourself feel pampered.)

❖ **MINT:** Members of the mint family such as peppermint and spearmint are also popular remedies for nausea. (For some people, though, peppermint can make nausea worse, because it may relax the lower esophageal sphincter and can thus potentially increase heartburn.) If you're on the go and can't stop to brew a cup of tea, try chewing a piece of mint gum or eating a small mint candy. Alternatively, you can carry a cotton ball with a drop of peppermint oil on it to sniff when you feel queasy; slip it in a sealable baggie or in an empty pill bottle to carry it without staining your clothes or bag.

❖ **CHAMOMILE:** Chamomile tea is a general relaxant. It helps you fall asleep and eases nausea and stomach discomfort. If you have an allergy or sensitivity to ragweed, be very cautious trying chamomile tea, as it is a member of the same family. If you already take chamomile with no ill effect, you should be all right to continue using it throughout your pregnancy. As chamomile is a very mild emmenagogue (i.e., can encourage uterine contractions), drink no more than one to two cups per day. Avoid using the oil, as it is a highly concentrated form of the plant.

❖ **RASPBERRY LEAF (*Rubus idaeus*):** Use with care during pregnancy; raspberry leaf acts as a uterine stimulant in high doses. Your medical professional may direct you to take raspberry leaf tea in the final month of your pregnancy to tone the uterus, which aids in labor.

Self-medicating can be a dangerous thing, but some health professionals will direct you to take teas or capsules of the following herbs near the end of your pregnancy to help prepare for labor. If you are interested in reading more about the safe use of herbs throughout pregnancy, a good resource is Susun S. Weed's *Wise Woman Herbal for the Childbearing Year*.

Herbs to Use with Care and Herbs to Avoid

There are some very familiar herbs that can be dangerous to a pregnant woman. Granted, you'll probably not miscarry if you eat a cookie that has a trace of cinnamon in it, but if you do a brisk rubdown with a liniment containing cinnamon oil to stimulate circulation you may have a problem on your hands.

Generally, this information applies to ingesting the herb, specifically self-medicating with it. Never ingest oils unless specifically instructed to do so by your medical professional, and then take them at the precise dosage and in the precise manner instructed. Oils are highly concentrated versions of the plant and can cause grave illness and death in an adult, let alone a fetus. Most of these herbs are contraindicated because they are uterine stimulants, which can trigger premature labor in high doses and may cause birth defects. Please use this information responsibly.

Herbs qualify as medicine, so if you are concerned about taking them internally please consult your medical professional. Essential oils are concentrated essences of the herb, and they are even more dangerous than the herb itself. Use them very carefully or discontinue your use of them altogether while pregnant. See Chapter 6 for a list of essential oils that are safe to use during pregnancy. For information regarding the use of herbs in ritual or spellcraft, see Chapter 5.

These warnings don't expire as soon as you give birth. Most of these herbs should be avoided while nursing as well. Check with your medical professional or lactation consultant.

This is not an exhaustive list; it simply includes the herbs that are likely to be on your kitchen shelves or in your magical cabinet that you use for potions or infusions. For a more complete reference, please consult a reliable medical herbal guide.

Herbs to avoid or to use with care during pregnancy include:

❖ **ALOE (*A. vera*):** External use only; do not ingest.

❖ **ANGELICA (*Angelica archangelica*):** Use with care; uterine stimulant in high doses.

❖ **ANISE (*Pimpinella anisum*):** Use with care; uterine stimulant in high doses.

❖ **ARNICA (*Arnica montana*):** The homeopathic ointment or gel is dilute enough that it should be all right to use in order to speed up the healing of bumps and bruises. Do not take arnica internally unless directed to do so by a licensed homeopath, as it is a uterine stimulant at high doses.

❖ **BASIL (*Ocimum basilicum*):** Use with care; uterine stimulant at high doses. Regular use as seasoning in cooking should be fine. May affect lactation. Do not use the oil while pregnant.

❖ **BLACK COHOSH (*Cimicifuga racemosus*):** Uterine stimulant; do not use during pregnancy. Your medical professional may instruct you to take black cohosh during labor, or to induce labor.

❖ **BLUE COHOSH (*Caulophyllum thalictroides*):** Uterine stimulant; do not use during pregnancy. Your medical professional may instruct you to take blue cohosh during labor, or to induce labor.

❖ **CELERY SEED (*Apium graveolens dulce*):** Use with care; uterine stimulant at high doses. Regular use as seasoning in cooking should be fine.

❖ **CINNAMON (*Cinnamomum zeylanicum*):** Use with care; uterine stimulant at high doses. Regular use as seasoning in cooking should be fine. Do not use the essential oil while pregnant.

❖ **CLOVE (*Syzygium aromaticum*):** Use with caution; uterine stimulant at high doses. The oil may be included as a component of a massage oil during labor.

❖ **COMFREY (*Symphytum officinale*):** Do not take comfrey internally during pregnancy.

❖ **DONG QUAI (*Angelica polymorpha* var. *sinensis*):** Avoid during pregnancy; uterine stimulant and emmenagogue.

❖ **FENNEL (*Foeniculum vulgare*):** Use with care; uterine stimulant at high doses. Regular use as seasoning in cooking should be fine. Do not use the oil during pregnancy.

❖ **FENUGREEK (*Trigonella foenum-graecum*):** Use with care; uterine stimulant at high doses. Regular use as seasoning in cooking should be fine.

❖ **FEVERFEW (*Tanacetum parthenium*):** Avoid during pregnancy; uterine stimulant.

❖ **GOLDENSEAL (*Hydrastis canadensis*):** Avoid during pregnancy; uterine stimulant. May be used during labor.

❖ **HOREHOUND (*Marrubium vulgare*):** Use with care; uterine stimulant at high doses. Regular use in cough drops and cough syrup should be fine.

❖ **JUNIPER (*Juniperus communis*):** Avoid during pregnancy; uterine stimulant. The oil may be a component of a massage oil during labor.

❖ **MARJORAM (*Origanum vulgare*):** Use with care during pregnancy; uterine stimulant at high doses. Regular use as seasoning in cooking should be fine. Do not use the oil while pregnant.

❖ **MISTLETOE (*Viscum album*):** Avoid during pregnancy; uterine stimulant and may cause birth defects.

❖ **MUGWORT (*Artemisia vulgaris*):** Avoid during pregnancy and breastfeeding; uterine stimulant.

❖ **MYRRH (*Commiphora molmol*):** Use with care during pregnancy; uterine stimulant at high doses.

❖ **NUTMEG (*Myristica* spp.):** Avoid during pregnancy; hallucinogenic and may cause birth defects. Regular use as seasoning in cooking should be fine.

❖ **OREGANO (*Origanum* × *marjoricum, O. onites*):** Use with care during pregnancy; uterine stimulant at high doses. Regular use as seasoning in cooking should be fine. Do not use the oil while pregnant.

❖ **PARSLEY (*Petroselinum crispum*):** Use with care during pregnancy; uterine stimulant at high doses. Regular use as seasoning in cooking should be fine.

❖ **PASSIONFLOWER (*Passiflora incarnata*):** Use with care during pregnancy; uterine stimulant at high doses.

❖ **PENNYROYAL (*Hedeoma pulegioides, Mentha pulegium*):** Avoid during pregnancy and breastfeeding; uterine stimulant.

❖ **ROSEMARY (*Rosmarinus officinalis*):** Use with care during pregnancy; uterine stimulant at high doses. Regular use as seasoning in cooking should be fine. Do not use the oil while pregnant.

❖ **RUE (*Ruta graveolens*):** Avoid during pregnancy and breast-feeding; uterine stimulant.

❖ **SAFFRON (*Crocus sativa*):** Use with care during pregnancy; uterine stimulant at high doses. Regular use as seasoning in cooking should be fine.

❖ **SAGE (*Salvia officinalis*):** Use with care during pregnancy; uterine stimulant at high doses. Regular use as seasoning in cooking should be fine. Do not use the oil while pregnant.

❖ **THYME (*Thymus vulgaris*):** Use with care during pregnancy; uterine stimulant at high doses. Regular use as seasoning in cooking should be fine. Do not use the oil while pregnant.

❖ **VERVAIN (*Verbena officinalis*):** Use with care during pregnancy; uterine stimulant at high doses.

❖ **WORMWOOD (*Artemisia absinthium*):** Avoid during pregnancy; uterine stimulant and may cause birth defects. Also avoid when breastfeeding.

❖ **YARROW (*Achillea millefolium*):** Use with care during pregnancy; uterine stimulant at high doses.

Common sense should govern your use of herbs during pregnancy, as it should any other time. If you are ever concerned or undecided about using an herb, be it in the form of a tea, incense, essential oil, or seasoning, err on the side of caution and do not use it. Consult with a medical professional or a licensed herbalist for more information.

Chapter 5
Responsible Energy Work

A large part of the neo-pagan spiritual path concerns itself with working with energy through ritual and spellwork, as well as simple everyday awareness of energy flow. While this work is undeniably strengthening on the whole, it also opens you up to dangers when you are pregnant that you may not have considered.

You should be aware of what kind of energy you're working with and how you use it. Consider carefully the energy you channel or handle while you are pregnant. Just because you can handle it doesn't mean the baby can. Just as the baby would absorb the alcohol from your bloodstream if you drank, and even a small amount can have an impact because the fetus is small and light compared to you, so, too, will the baby feel the effects of any energy you channel. This chapter will look at how to practice rituals, spellwork, and other interactions with energy in ways that are safe for both you and your unborn baby.

Energy Work While Pregnant

Being aware of how you handle energy and how you react in strong-energy situations is important in general when you walk a neo-pagan path and practice ritual, but this kind of self-awareness is crucial while you are pregnant. Just as your physical and emotional bodies go through changes that force you to constantly re-evaluate how you move and react, so, too, does your personal energy shift, reflecting those physical, emotional, and mental changes through which you progress. The child you carry is especially sensitive to the energy that you use and interact with. In general, it is important to be aware that heavy, hard, sudden, and/or fast-moving energy can harm the baby. Energy can also indirectly harm the fetus by affecting you in a negative way. If the energy ends up being too much for you in any respect, it can trigger labor or miscarriage, just as any other sudden physical, emotional, or stress-related shock can do.

It's best to be cautious. And many neo-pagan mothers-to-be instinctively engage in this kind of self-regulation when it comes to ritual or spellwork, choosing to not participate in rituals that work with energy they do not feel comfortable with, even if they would have been comfortable with the energy or ritual focus before their pregnancy.

As part of your responsible magical practice while pregnant, limit participation in deep rituals such as initiations, elevations, and so forth, both for yourself and in facilitating them for other people. These types of rituals trigger intense change on multiple levels and are life-changing for the individuals undergoing them and leading them. You can imagine how deeply the fetus may be affected.

Aspecting

If you aspect as part of your practice or worship, you may wish to limit or forgo the technique while pregnant. Aspecting is the powerful and challenging technique by which an individual calls into him or herself another entity, usually a deity but sometimes another essence, and serves as a host for that entity for the purposes of communication, communion, wisdom, insight, or healing, among other things. If you intend to aspect while carrying a baby, think carefully about the deity you intend to aspect while pregnant. When you aspect, you function as the host for that deity's energy and personality. Your fetus also serves as cohost for the deity, or is totally enveloped by the deity's energy. Think of how aspecting affects you, how it leaves its mark for a period of time. Then consider how much longer your fetus will carry the effects of the aspecting.

If you wish to continue aspecting, think about working with a mother goddess, perhaps one of the mother goddesses from Chapter 3. Even then, limit your time aspecting, and always aspect with a companion present who can monitor you. (This is sound advice for anyone at any time, even when not pregnant, but all the more important when your energy is changing on a day-to-day basis and you're not sure of how your energy will respond to hosting deity today.)

If you wish to begin aspecting a specific mother goddess, perhaps the one you have chosen to work with throughout your pregnancy, do as much research as possible on that goddess before aspecting her. If you decide to aspect Cybele, for example, bear in mind that her devotees used to honor her by participating in orgiastic and sometimes violent ritual, and this may have an echo of sorts when you invite her in.

Grounding and Centering

In pregnancy, your personal energy changes. How it changes and to what extent it will change depends completely on how you and your baby interact with each other on an energy level, and on how your body and spirit respond instinctively to pregnancy. As noted elsewhere, it will likely also be different from pregnancy to pregnancy: You can't necessarily rely on your last pregnancy to predict how your energy will change during your next pregnancy.

Because things change so drastically and without warning, it's important to maintain a solid and reliable connection to the energy of the earth. The earth is the most constant source of energy we have: It is always there and always accessible. During pregnancy there will be times when you suddenly feel tired, or overwhelmed, or wobbly, or hyped up, or buzzed. Grounding helps you balance emotions, helps you with your physical balance and your physical comfort, and helps you stabilize your energy levels.

The basic uses of grounding are:

❖ **TO REBALANCE:** This is very useful with constantly fluctuating emotions and physical sensations of pregnancy.

❖ **TO ENERGIZE:** Drawing energy up from the earth helps refresh your own personal energy when you're tired or feeling low or listless.

There are dozens and dozens of basic how-to descriptions of centering and grounding available in a variety of websites and books, including my own *Spellcrafting, Wicca: A Modern Practioner's Guide,* and *The Green Witch*. A brief guide to centering and grounding is included here for the sake of completeness; many of the rituals described in this book call for the use of these techniques.

Before beginning the grounding sequence, you should use the technique called centering. Fundamentally, centering encompasses drawing your personal energy into your energy center before proceeding with your chosen activity. Your energy center is a place that serves as the seat of your personal energy, often a chakra such as the solar plexus. (For more information on your personal energy center, see *Spellcrafting* or *Wicca: A Modern Practioner's Guide*.) Centering can be done as a first step before grounding, or whenever you wish to focus your energy if you feel scattered or weakened by directing your energy in too many different directions at once.

Once you have centered, you can then ground:

1. Focus on your solar plexus. (This is in fact a chakra, one of many energy centers in the body.)

2. Visualize your solar plexus pulsating with a sparkling light.

3. Imagine a root made of this sparkling light growing from your solar plexus down through your body toward the ground. Visualize this root extending down through the building into the earth below.

4. Visualize the root of light connecting with the energy of the earth. Then allow the earth's energy to rise up through this root to your solar plexus and from there spread through your body.

5. When you feel that it is time to disconnect, visualize the root disconnecting from the earth's energy and being drawn back up to your solar plexus.

It's important to note that you don't have to disconnect from the earth's energy. You can remain plugged in to the earth's energy at all times with no ill effect. In fact, it provides you with the physical stability mentioned earlier, and also keeps you in touch with calming, soothing energy that can refresh you if you require it, or it can shunt off excess energy if you become too agitated.

It's particularly important to remember while pregnant not to use too much of your own personal energy to power spells or energy work. Your energy is involved in doing other things, so although you may feel as if you have energy to spare at certain points, it's there for a reason. Drawing too much of it away may deprive the child of the energy it requires for its own sustenance or protection. If you need to use energy for something, make a habit of centering and grounding in order to draw that energy up from the ground instead of using your own personal energy.

Preparing for Ritual

As every neo-pagan path is different, this book makes no assumptions as to what you may or may not customarily do in ritual, or even that you do ritual at all. As a result, you may have noticed that most of the rituals in this book direct you to "prepare sacred space as per your customary practice." Essentially, this means that you should use your standard preparation and opening for ritual if you have one. If you don't, this chapter will offer you basic structures to use.

If you prefer to work in space that has been blessed, but not in a formal circle, refer to the following section on creating sacred space. If you wish to work in a formally delineated space with a bit more structure to it, refer to the following basic circle-cast.

Every once in a while a ritual will direct you specifically to use a formal circle. This is because the ritual itself requires a more concrete formal space to protect you or to contain the energy with which you're working. Other times, sacred space is all that is required, so you may choose to use a circle or sacred space as you desire. Ultimately, the most important thing to do before any of these rituals or spells is to set apart your area as sacred space, delineated from the everyday in some fashion, which helps you focus mentally and spiritually by allowing you to walk through a familiar (or soon-to-be familiar) process.

Circle or Sacred Space?

A circle is a formally defined temple in which the everyday world and the world of the gods meet. This place is where you can connect with the gods in a ritual fashion. A circle is cast or raised as a ceremonial way of crafting a temple in which to commune or worship.

Sacred space, on the other hand, is an informal area that has been purified and blessed, cleansed of any negative or unsupportive energy, but not formally separated from the surrounding environment. Nor does it have a boundary that will keep negative or other energy away.

You may feel more comfortable creating a formal circle in which to work the rituals in this book, or you may prefer the simpler sacred space. Your desires or needs may vary according to how you feel that day or depending on how formal you wish your observance to be.

Creating Sacred Space

There are three basic steps to creating sacred space:

1. **Cleansing:** physically removing detritus from the area
2. **Purifying:** eliminating negative energy from the area
3. **Blessing:** bringing in positive energy to support your goal

If you'd like to create a basic sacred space in which to work, you can do so by circling your space with physical representations of the four elements while visualizing each element, leaving a trail of charged energy as it passes through the air. You can even turn in place and raise the element to the four cardinal directions, visualizing the energy of the element reaching out from your central point, pushing away any unwanted energy.

Here are some suggestions to use alone or in combination as you create sacred space:

❖ Sweep the area with a broom reserved for spiritual use. As you do, visualize the energy of the area being purified of anything negative, muddy, or stale.

❖ Carry a lit incense stick around the space you intend to use. As you do, visualize the energy of the area being purified as in the previous suggestion.

❖ Light a candle and visualize the light reaching outward and pushing the energy before it to illumine the space. Carry it around the space, or leave it in the center.

❖ Finally, take a small cup or bowl of water and sprinkle a pinch of salt into it. Dip your fingers into the water, then flick them outward to shake off the drops from your fingertips, using the water to further bless the space.

Sacred space doesn't have to be dismissed or undone in any way when you are finished. The energy of the surrounding environment will gradually flow through it and return it to its everyday status.

Casting a Circle

What is termed a *circle* is in fact a sphere of energy that protects you from all directions. Here's a very basic description of how to raise a simple circle:

1. Stand in the center of the space in which you intend to work. Breathe deeply a few times to relax yourself and to focus. Center and ground.

2. Draw earth energy up through your connection to the earth.

3. Lift your hand and point at the border you intend to define with your circle. Allow the earth energy you have collected in your energy center to flow down your arm to your hand. Standing in place, begin to turn clockwise.

4. As you turn, project the energy out through your fingers to draw a line along the border of your space. Will this energy to form a barrier between your workspace and the world beyond.

5. Turn and project this energy until you have returned to the point at which you began. You will have described a complete circle with the energy.

6. Take a moment to visualize the circle of energy growing taller and curving up over your head until all the sides meet above you, so that you are standing within a dome of energy. Now visualize the edges of the circle reaching down below you, meeting far beneath your feet, so that you are standing within a complete sphere of energy.

What you do with the circle once it's there is up to you. You can just move on to your ritual, or you may wish to do something along the lines described earlier in the sacred space directions to purify and consecrate the circle with the four elements. Or you may wish to move on formally, invoking the elements and inviting deity to share your temple space, if this is part of your customary practice. If you're looking for other information about the basic circle-cast with no religious overtone, you can refer to *Spellcrafting*. If you're Wiccan, you can delve into more detail about sacred space and circles in *Wicca: A Modern Practioner's Guide*. Most introductory Wiccan texts include instructions on how to raise a basic circle.

To take down or dissolve your circle, reverse the steps: Visualize the sphere shrinking back down into a simple line of energy, then extend your hand and turn counterclockwise in place, gathering the circle's energy back into your hand. Allow the energy to flow up your arm and through your energy center, then back down to the earth through your connection. Center and ground again to make sure that you've shaken off any excess energy. If you feel wobbly or dizzy, you may have shunted some of your own personal energy down into the earth along with the circle's energy; ground and draw up earth energy again until you feel stabilized.

Altars, Workspaces, and Tools

Again, this book does not presume anything regarding your regular mode of operations. However, it is recommended that you have a basic altar setup for these rituals and spells if you do not already have one. This is because tools and elemental representations have energy that you can draw upon, thus further protecting yourself from overusing your own personal energy.

What constitutes a basic altar setup? Well, the bare essentials are the elemental representations—something physical to honor the four physical elements of earth, air, fire, and water, such as a dish of earth, incense, a candle, and a bowl of water—and perhaps a cloth to place on the surface you're using as an altar.

Common neo-pagan tools also include a knife, a wand, and a cup. These three tools are often associated with elements as well, with fire and air being assigned to blades and wands interchangeably, depending on the tradition or path, and the cup symbolizing water. Some neo-pagans use a combination of tools and elemental representations.

Sympathetic magic is something neo-pagans work with a lot. In this type of magic, a knife called an athame is sometimes used to symbolically cut or carve things. During your pregnancy, you may be more comfortable using a wand instead of an athame. A wand has no edge to it, and thus symbolically may be safer to use than an edged weapon, particularly if you are concerned about miscarrying. Many cultures possess folk wisdom relating to the ill effects the energy of sharp or bladed objects can have upon the fetus.

Basic Review of Meditation

There are plenty of books out there on meditation, so there's no point in covering the topic in depth. Chances are good that you already meditate in some form or another. So here's just a quick review.

There are four basic aspects to successful meditation:

❖ **A QUIET ENVIRONMENT:** Lots of noise tends to distract you from your meditative focus. Visual distractions like a window to a busy street, or a TV on with the sound off, or people walking through your space are equally detrimental to meditation. Choose a quiet place where you'll be able to meditate undisturbed. (This is in no way meant to invalidate the experiences of those who can meditate on public transport at rush hour, but merely a recommendation for more successful meditation.)

❖ **CORRECT PHYSICAL POSITION:** Posture is important. Sitting uncomfortably will distract you from your meditative focus, as well as risking physical damage. Use an upright chair and sit with your arms and legs uncrossed. You may want to place something under your feet to reduce the edge of the seat's pressure on the backs of your thighs. Sitting on the floor is fine, but be aware that if you cross your legs you may compromise the flow of blood through your legs when pregnant. Lying down is not usually a good idea, because it's a signal to your body and brain that you're ready to fall asleep. Certain meditations in this book direct you to lie down for them, however, due to the nature of the meditation.

❖ **A RELAXATION SEQUENCE:** It's hard to just sit down and drop into a deep meditation. You'll need some sort of sequence to get yourself into the right frame of mind and physical state for successful meditation. This can be a simple lighting of a candle or incense and some deep breathing with your eyes closed, or as complex as a set premeditation meditation, such as counting down from ten to one while imagining yourself walking down a staircase. The trick is to use the same sequence every time to facilitate attaining the right state.

❖ **A FOCUS:** A focus is some sort of mental device that allows you to keep your mind engaged and stops it from wandering around and chattering away at you. A focus can be a mantra, a thought or spoken phrase upon which to concentrate; a visual focus to look at; or a breathing pattern (see the following example).

These four things are commonly found within meditative practice. They can be as casual or formal as you like, but each of them benefits the meditative experience in some way.

Breathing Meditation

When you're pregnant, you need a lot more of everything: sleep, water, nutrients, oxygen, and so forth. Your body steps up the pace of everything, making more blood and using energy to grow and nurture another life and body, safely protected inside yours.

As your body shifts and grows, you need to refocus your physical posture and movement in order to accommodate the new mass and weight distribution. The same is true of your breathing technique.

Engaging in breathing meditation is a simple way to relax and rebalance your personal energy. The point of breathing meditation is to allow yourself the opportunity to relax, to allow your body the opportunity to absorb more oxygen, and to allow your mind the quiet time and space it requires to deal with the changes and stress of daily life.

It may seem counterintuitive to actively practice breathing; after all, it's part of an automatic system, an action your body takes whether you will it to or not. However, by focusing on your breath, you allow yourself to become more mindful of your own body, the energy you use maintaining it, and the respect you owe your physical temple.

The concept of the physical body being the house for the spiritual temple is an interesting one to examine in conjunction with breathing meditation. You can think of breathing meditation as a method by which the physical temple is cleansed, with exhalations sweeping it clean of the negative energy that clutters up the space and inhalation purifying the space with blessed pure air.

By meditating on an unconscious action like breathing, you can draw attention to the functions of your body that carry on without your conscious attention, such as the nourishment and incubation of the child growing within that physical temple. Furthermore, by actively focusing on an unconscious action like breathing, you can influence your body's well-being. You can breathe faster, slower, more deeply, more shallowly, and by doing so observe a direct response in your body.

In breathing meditation, one usually focuses on slowing down one's breathing so that the physical body relaxes and releases tension. As a rule in breathing meditation, breathe naturally, and allow the breath flowing in and out to become the focus of your attention. Don't actively think "in, out, in, out"; rather, observe the breath flowing. Try breathing in through your nose and exhaling through your mouth.

If you find your mind wandering while you breathe, and you have difficulty focusing simply on your breath as it flows in and out of your lungs, you can count while you breathe. Try breathing in to a count of four, pausing for a count of two, then exhaling for a count of four. By counting, you provide your mind with this simple and repetitive task to occupy it in order to allow your body to relax.

Your medical professional or prenatal workshop leader will probably talk to you about using breathing patterns to help you remain relaxed throughout labor. Focusing on your breathing allows you to redirect your attention from worrying about what's happening in your body, as well as providing you with an easy method of relaxing the natural tension that develops, which can sometimes affect the productivity of the uterine contractions. Too, some women focus so much on the physical process that they forget to breathe, so breathing patterns and breathing meditation can help you remember to take in the oxygen necessary to keep you conscious and functioning at the best level possible.

Working with Shields

If you haven't worked with personal shields before, now is the time to address this important issue. Personal shields are some of the most fundamental ways you have of protecting yourself. Much as you instinctively protect the child you carry within your body in response to physical threat by curling your body around your womb or cradling your abdomen in your arms, personal shields can protect the fetus from ambient energy, attack, and so forth.

Here is a basic outline to create a personal shield that can deflect energy, filter energy, or at the very least warn you that something's up:

1. Center and ground. (See instructions earlier in this chapter.)

2. Draw energy up from the ground into your personal energy center.

3. Visualize this energy forming a ball. Visualize this ball growing steadily, expanding outward in all directions until you are standing within a sphere made of energy.

4. Visualize this sphere hardening and taking on a tangible surface that can stop energy from passing through it toward you.

Some people like to visualize the exterior of their shield as a mirror, bouncing energy away from them, or as flames destroying any negative energy that attempts to make its way through the shield. Others prefer to leave the shield as a warning system, a kind of extension of their personal senses or awareness that serves to alert them to shifts in energy.

Additionally, you may wish to curtail your interaction with indefinable or unrecognizable energy. If you're not familiar with a certain type of energy you encounter, either in ritual or in the everyday world, then let discretion be the better part of valor: Avoid it, strengthen your shields, and don't expose the baby to it.

Using Supplies with Caution

In general, your basic supplies ought to be safe to continue using during pregnancy in your rituals and spellwork. However, be sure to read the ingredients list on teas and incenses carefully. Make sure the wicks of the candles you use don't have lead centers. (You should be doing these things on a regular basis anyway, but now it's even more important.) Wash your hands thoroughly and frequently after working with tools and supplies.

There are certain supplies, though, to which you should pay particular attention in using when you are pregnant: herbs and essential oils. Contraindicated herbs are generally classified as such because there is no concrete proof that they are safe.

Limit or discontinue use of essential oils completely in your spellcraft and rituals. Essential oils are highly concentrated essences of plants, and a drop or two of certain oils can be enough to harm a full-grown adult if misused, let alone a fetus. If you are concerned about the safety of your essential oils, use fragrance oils instead. There are some people who feel that fragrance oils carry no energy associated with the actual plant essence, but in the system of magical correspondences and symbolism, they do. (Refer to the lists in Chapter 4 to familiarize yourself with the herbs and oils that are contraindicated for use during pregnancy.) Symbolism is what allows us to use a picture or sketch of something to represent the real item. In this way, a fragrance oil that smells somewhat like the original plant is a symbol of the real thing, even if it is created artificially. A fragrance oil can be much safer than the essential oil, despite its nonnatural origins.

Also limit your use of herbs in spellcraft and ritual. Beware of burning them in incenses; discontinue brewing and drinking potions while pregnant unless they are approved by your doctor (lavender, mint, or chamomile infusions in moderation, for example). Taking herbal teas or herbal supplements constitutes taking medication, and many medications are proscribed during pregnancy for their unknown effects upon the fetus. As contraindicated herbs are usually classified as such for self-medication and internal use, handling herbs for herbal sachets or spell bags or powders is usually all right, but pay special attention to those herbs that are contraindicated or to be used with care during pregnancy (such as mugwort or sage). Take extra care handling them in ways you may be used to handling them, such as smudging with them. In fact, it's better to be safe rather than sorry, so try using one of these techniques: invoking the herb's energy without a physical sample of it there, or replacing the contraindicated herb with a magical substitution. Here's how to preform these techniques.

Technique One: Invoke the Herb's Energy

Much the way you can invoke an element without a physical representation of it present, you can call upon the correspondences of the herb to add to your spell or ritual without actually having the herb present. For example, if a spell you were casting called for angelica as one of the ingredients in an herbal sachet for protection, you could hold your hands over the otherwise completed sachet and say:

> *Angelica,*
> *Herb of protection,*
> *I call upon you now to lend your energy to my spell.*
> *Lend me your aid this day.*

Angelica, I honor you.
Thank you for your gift.
So may it be.

Technique Two: Magical Substitution

First of all, to substitute effectively, look at the purpose for the herb's inclusion in your spell or recipe. Is the recipe geared toward protection? Try substituting another herb you personally associate with protection that has a similar energy to the herb you wish to replace. All the standard advice regarding substitutions applies: Don't substitute with an herb with which you are unfamiliar; don't substitute with an herb to which you have demonstrated a sensitivity; don't substitute with an herb that doesn't play well with the other ingredients you're using. And of course, don't substitute with an herb that's also on the list of herbs to avoid during pregnancy.

The following is a list of herbs that you should be careful using magically while pregnant and suggested magical substitutions.

❖ **MISTLETOE:** For protection, substitute rose. For fertility, substitute myrtle.

❖ **MUGWORT:** For psychic powers, substitute magnolia or carnation. For divination, substitute daisy.

❖ **WORMWOOD:** For protection, substitute cedar. For purification/cleansing/banishing, substitute frankincense or garlic.

❖ **NUTMEG:** For justice, substitute John the Conqueror.

❖ **SAGE:** Do not burn. For purification, use lavender or cedar.

Additionally, if from previous experience you know yourself to be sensitive to the energy of certain herbs or oils that aren't on the contraindicated list, limit or discontinue the use of them while pregnant as well. And above all, trust your instincts. If a spell or ritual calls for a certain herb or oil, and you have a strong resistance to using it that may have no logical foundation, find a replacement for it.

Personal Energy and Pregnancy

Your personal energy changes over the course of your pregnancy. Personal energy changes all the time, of course, but during your pregnancy your personal energy will alter and shift in a more marked fashion. This change can produce unexpected effects in spell and ritual, as well as destabilizing you in meditation and so forth if you expect a certain response from your energy to a specific stimulus, and you get a stronger or weaker response, or another response entirely.

On a very basic level, your energy will no longer be entirely your own: There is energy produced by the growth and development of the fetus to take into account. This energy shifts over time as well, as the fetus itself is constantly changing.

In addition to this, your energy kicks into high gear, for you are literally in the throes of creation. Creation uses and produces a lot of energy. Emotion also produces energy, and during pregnancy emotion runs high, as is perfectly normal and understandable. Interestingly enough, high emotion is also an observable effect of personal energy shifting, so these two things are correlated. Chapter 6 will help you explore and navigate these physical, emotional, and energy shifts.

Chapter 6

Preparing for Change

It is physically obvious that pregnancy is a time of change, but it's also a time for emotional change. Unfortunately, the emotional changes aren't as well mapped out as the physical transformation. And while you can get used to the physical difference, it's harder to get a grip on the emotional changes when they vary daily, or several times daily.

This chapter is divided into two parts. The first part looks at the emotional changes that occur during pregnancy and offers techniques to help explore them and deal with them. The second part looks at how to handle your response to the changes in your physical body.

Dealing with Emotional Changes

While some of the emotional changes you will encounter during pregnancy stem from the very real fluctuation in hormonal production and balance, much of the emotional upheaval is linked to the stress caused by fear of the unknown. And this sort of stress isn't the type that can be handled with a cup of chamomile tea and a good night's sleep: The emotional stress of pregnancy goes much deeper than that.

Ironically, part of the emotional stress is derived from the emotional ups and downs themselves. You may perceive yourself reacting in a more emotional fashion to a situation that you know you would have responded to differently before your pregnancy, and you may fear that you are acting irrationally. You may wonder if you've changed permanently, or how drastic and how consistent these shifts and changes will be.

It's important to remember that every woman responds to the chemical and hormonal fluctuations of pregnancy in a different way. Each and every way, however, is valid, and deserves careful and considerate support. It's important to take your needs seriously.

The physical changes can wear you down: dealing with fatigue, nausea, and a body whose shape is shifting daily. Pregnancy also demands a great deal of mental and emotional energy, making everyday life a challenge.

Some of the emotional stress comes from the uncertainty about the future, which makes perfect sense, as one never knows precisely what to expect when one completes a rite of passage into a new role. You can theoretically understand your future responsibilities, but you cannot know how they will impact you psychologically. Whether consciously or subconsciously, you may worry about things such as:

- ❖ What will change in my life?
- ❖ How will I respond to this new set of responsibilities?
- ❖ What will happen to my relationship with my partner? With my parents? With my siblings? With my friends?

Allow yourself the time to think about your pregnancy. Ask yourself on a regular basis how you feel about being pregnant, how you feel about parenting, and how you feel about your changing role in your immediate family and in society.

Something that may come up is a sense of regret, even if you're thrilled about your pregnancy and eagerly looking forward to your baby and your new role. Regret and a sense of sorrow are a natural part of transitioning through a rite of passage, for you are in a sense grieving for your past life. It's perfectly normal to be emotional about, and sometimes wish to return to, your previous child-free state. In fact, this wave of emotion will probably occur again at some point during labor. Acknowledging and allowing yourself to feel these emotions without judgment is important. It's all right to feel the way you do, no matter what those feelings may be. Every feeling during pregnancy is valid, because it's a unique expression of yourself and how you're integrating the facts and future of your pregnancy into your psyche. Your emotional response to your pregnancy at any given time is important and legitimate.

Keeping a Pregnancy Journal

The point of a spiritual journal is to keep a record of your spiritual journey: how you feel, the experiences you have while meditating, and the details and results of your rituals and spells. Your journal also serves as a place to note down research and thoughts. The value of keeping a spiritual journal is rarely immediately apparent, beyond the desire to capture something meaningful or fleeting for posterity. The true value lies in being able to return to your past journaling to examine it for themes, rhythms, and symbolism pertinent to your later work.

In keeping a pregnancy journal, you not only have the opportunity to note down physical changes, but emotional and spiritual changes as well. Whether you choose to journal daily or weekly, your record offers you the chance to preserve your spiritual journey.

Choose a new journal, one that you will use for this pregnancy only. Make sure you mark the dates clearly in it so that if you need to reference it at a later point you'll be able to easily find the time you're looking for.

You might choose to include all your spells and rituals in this journal, whether they have something specific to do with your pregnancy or not, or you might want to keep a journal that is focused solely on pregnancy-related issues; the choice is up to you. For the sake of completeness, you should journal your spells and rituals in your regular magical record book as usual, and make a copy to insert in the appropriate place in your pregnancy journal.

It's best to use a sturdy notebook, hardcover or softcover, with a bound spine. Coils tend to get caught on things, and loose-leaf paper in a binder can get shuffled, torn, or lost. Look for a notebook with a pleasing color or image on it, one that calms you or makes you think of harmony, serenity, nature, motherhood, family, or the Goddess—whatever speaks to you as right for your personal pregnancy journal.

A beautiful way to dedicate this journal is to write a book blessing for it. A book blessing is a kind of written spell that seals your intent into the book. Take some time to create one of your own, or use this one:

> *As I travel along this sacred path,*
> *May the words and images I inscribe herein*
> *Reflect the Divine energy I carry within me.*
> *Throughout my voyage of discovery,*
> *May I move in harmony with the world around me.*
> *May I spread fertile, blossoming, prosperous energy*
> *As I journey hand in hand with the Goddess.*
> *As I write, so may it be.*

The following is a full ritual with which to dedicate your spiritual pregnancy journal.

Ritual for Blessing Your Pregnancy Journal

Before this ritual, choose the book you will use for your pregnancy journal. If you like, choose a pen to use solely for writing in this journal; you can bless the pen during the ritual too. Have ready your book blessing as well (see example in previous section), unless you prefer to create a blessing extemporaneously during the ritual itself.

The candle should be large enough that it can burn throughout this ritual and have plenty left over, so that you can burn it each time that you write in your pregnancy journal (see the ritual for journaling in the next section). A fifteen-hour votive is ideal. If you journal a lot, and the candle burns down, you can bless a new one to use while journaling.

YOU WILL NEED

- Sandalwood incense (or lavender or violet)
- Censer
- Frankincense oil
- White candle (or pale yellow)
- Candleholder
- Matches or a lighter

- A blank journal
- A pen
- A copy of your book blessing (optional)
- Candle snuffer (optional; you can use your fingers)

DIRECTIONS

1. Cast a circle as per your customary method.

2. Invoke deity. You may call both the God and the Goddess to be present in your circle, or the Goddess only. If you work with a specific goddess, you may invoke her.

3. Light the sandalwood incense and place it in the censer, saying:
   Sacred wood, I ask for your blessing.

4. Take a dab of frankincense oil on your finger and anoint the candle, saying:
   I bless you in the name of the Mother Goddess.

5. Light the candle, saying:
   Sacred flame, I ask for your blessing.
   When I come again to light you,
   Be for me a symbol of hope and serenity.
   Help me to be open to all the layers of meaning
   In the thoughts I write down.
   Help me to be open to this experience,
   To learn from it,
   And be enriched by it.
   As I will,
   So may it be.

6. Take a dab of frankincense oil upon your finger and touch the four corners of the cover of the blank journal, saying:

   Book, I bless you in the name of the Goddess.

7. If you wish, you may anoint the spine and back cover as well. (At this point, if you have chosen to bless a pen with which to write in your spiritual pregnancy journal, you may anoint it as well, saying: *Pen, I bless you in the name of the Goddess.*)

8. Take the blank journal in your hands. Center and ground, and close your eyes. Breathe deeply and slowly draw earth energy up through your grounding. Let it flow down your hands and absorb into the book. Say:

   Journal, I call upon you
   To be for me a haven,
   A place where thought and experience
   Meld to become sacred guides.
   Goddess, I call upon you to bless this journal.
   May I be blessed each time I open it.
   With every page I fill, may I draw closer to you,
   And closer to that mystery of life and birth
   That so captures the hearts of humanity.

9. Open the front cover and write your name, the date, and any other information you wish to record on the first page. If you'd like, copy your book blessing onto the page as well. If you wish you may take another dab of oil and anoint the book blessing.

10. Turn the page, write the date again, and make your very first entry in your spiritual pregnancy journal. Write down how you feel about learning that you are pregnant, your hopes and fears, your goals, your thoughts on becoming a mother.

11. When you are done, close the book and say:

    I thank you for sharing your energy.

> *Incense and candle, book and pen,*
> *Blessings upon you.*

12. Use the candle snuffer (if using) to extinguish the candle; otherwise pinch it out with your fingers. Set the candle aside to be lit again when you next write in your journal (see the following ritual).

13. Thank and release deity, and take down your circle.

Journaling Ritual

This ritual echoes the ritual to bless your journal. It's meant to create a sense of consistency and familiarity in order to enhance your journaling experience. A familiar sequence and repeated use of ritual tools also helps you make the most of your journaling time by getting you into the correct headspace in a shorter amount of time, very like a psychological trigger.

This ritual is less formal than the previous one, however. It is not necessary to create a formal circle every time you wish to journal, although if you wish to you certainly can do it. It is a good idea to create sacred space, however, for your journal is one of the methods through which you attune yourself to the Goddess, and sacred space provides a less cluttered atmosphere and energy in which to make that attunement.

YOU WILL NEED

- ❖ Sandalwood incense
- ❖ Censer
- ❖ White candle (candle from the previous ritual to bless your pregnancy journal)
- ❖ Candleholder
- ❖ Matches or a lighter
- ❖ Your journal and a pen
- ❖ Candle snuffer (optional)

DIRECTIONS

1. Create sacred space as per your customary practice.

2. Center and ground. Breathe deeply and calmly to relax your mind and body.

3. Light the incense. Light the candle. Breathe, focusing on the air flowing in and out of your lungs. Allow the scent of sandalwood and the candle flame to relax you and help you achieve the calm and open headspace for journaling.

4. Hold your journal in your hands or on your lap as you breathe. When you are ready to journal, open the book and take up your pen. If you like, you may say something such as:

   May the words I write
   Open my heart and spirit
   To the touch of the Goddess.

5. Write in your journal. When you are finished, close the book and say:

   I thank the Goddess for my words and thoughts.
   May I continue to be blessed by her love and care.

6. Extinguish the candle with the candle snuffer, pinch it out with your fingers, or blow it out. Allow the incense to burn down.

Think about the Perfect Mother

We all have a vision of the perfect mother. She's always calm, always serene; she smiles; she is never tired. She cares for her baby so well and so tenderly that it never cries and is never hungry, because she anticipates its needs. Her house is sparkling clean: There are no toys or magazines or coffee cups lying about, the kitchen is spotless, and there isn't a speck of dust on the ground. Every meal she serves to baby and family is home-cooked and delicious. She is completely and totally fulfilled by caring for her child.

She also doesn't exist.

You're going to kill yourself if you try to be the ideal mother.

Before you can address the artificial stereotype of the ideal mother, you'll need to dig into your subconscious and memories to pull out all the associations you have with the perfect mother.

YOU WILL NEED

- ❖ Candle
- ❖ Candleholder
- ❖ Incense
- ❖ Censer
- ❖ Matches or a lighter
- ❖ Your pregnancy journal
- ❖ Pen or pencil

DIRECTIONS

1. Create sacred space as per your usual practice.

2. Light the candle and the incense. Breathe deeply a few times to relax yourself.

3. Sit down with your journal and think about the concept of the ideal mother. What does she look like? What does she do? What does she not do?

4. Write down anything that comes into your head on the topic. Don't censor yourself or your thoughts—just allow them to rise, and write them down as they come. Do not dismiss anything because it sounds silly, shallow, or ridiculous. If the name of a specific person or deity comes to mind, write it down, but take some time before you conclude the exercise to figure out why

they represent the perfect mother to you. Write down the reasons. Some may already be on your list (excellent housekeeper, great cook, and so on).

5. When you feel you have listed all the things you associate with the ideal mother that you can, extinguish the candle and incense or allow them to burn out, as you wish.

6. Dismiss your sacred space as per your usual practice.

7. Over the next few days, more things may rise to your mind to add to your list. Write them down as they come to you.

This list serves a variety of purposes. First, it forces you to think of all the traits that you assign to the stereotype of the ideal mother. By writing them all down you can see how unrealistic they are. And by seeing the artificiality of the stereotype, you can begin to change how you expect yourself to behave once your baby has been born. You can be easier on yourself and redefine your expectations.

Remembering Who You Are

One of the most common fears among women who are expecting, whether they go so far as to define it or admit it to themselves or not, is that they will never again be the individual they are before the birth of their baby, that they will somehow lose the core of what makes them a unique individual. When the baby is born, will you become Mother so completely that you will no longer be Maureen, or Diane, or Beth?

It looks silly when it's put into words. Of course you don't stop being you. But the fear of loss of individuality isn't wholly rational.

It's a deep-seated fear that stems partially from the total and utter dependence an infant has upon its mother. The following journaling ritual will help you establish a baseline definition of your core self; carry this self-awareness with you through your pregnancy and after your baby is born.

YOU WILL NEED

- ❖ Candle
- ❖ Candleholder
- ❖ Incense
- ❖ Censer
- ❖ Matches or a lighter
- ❖ Your pregnancy journal
- ❖ Pen or pencil

DIRECTIONS

1. Create sacred space as per your usual practice.

2. Light the candle. Light the incense. Breathe deeply a few times to relax yourself.

3. Sit down with your journal and think about what defines you as an individual. What are your hobbies? Your likes and dislikes? How would you describe yourself to a stranger? If it helps, talk about yourself in the third person ("She is a kind and caring woman"). What are your accomplishments, your talents?

4. Write down anything that comes into your head. Don't censor yourself or your thoughts; just allow them to rise, and write them down as they come. Do not dismiss anything because it sounds silly, or shallow, or ridiculous. Be proud of who you are.

5. When you feel you have listed as many of the things as you can about what makes you you, go back and change any third-person statements to first-person statements. (For example, "She is a kind and caring woman" becomes "I am a kind and caring woman.")

6. Extinguish the candle and incense or allow them to burn out, as you wish.

7. Dismiss your sacred space as per your usual practice.

8. Over the next few days, more things may rise to your mind to add to your list. Write them down as they come to you.

This list serves a variety of purposes. First, it forces you to define yourself in words, instead of as a vague feeling. Seeing the words describing your attributes written down helps you comprehend that these things do not change; they are a part of you. Referring back to this list will also help ground your fears once the baby has been born and you need to look at who you are independently of the small creature that seems to be permanently attached to you.

Dealing with Physical Changes

During pregnancy, you have the opportunity to deeply explore the concept of the body being the physical temple that houses the spirit. On a day-to-day basis, the body is the temple that houses the spirit, your spirit. But while pregnant, you are housing two spirits (and before you argue about when a child is ensouled, let's just agree that it happens; so at some point there will be two spirits, one in the tiny child body forming and developing inside yours).

Honoring the body is a wonderful part of most neo-pagan paths. In pregnancy, the body can be further honored as a cradle of life, as the means by which life is incubated and brought forth, as a means through which we can participate in the ongoing cycle of life ourselves.

We become living incarnations of the life-giving aspect of the Goddess, the Great Mother herself.

Honoring Your Body

Your body is hard at work creating life. It is always a spiritual temple, but now more than ever it has become a thing of sacredness. Now more than ever, your body deserves your respect. First and foremost, honor your body by giving it the rest it requires. Rest and sleep are not the same thing. Rest allows you the mental, emotional, and spiritual space you need in order to stay functional; sleep gives you the physical break you need to survive.

Second, respect your body's needs, and feed and hydrate it regularly. We have a tendency to underestimate how much liquid we need on a daily basis even when we aren't pregnant. Drink at least six to eight 8-ounce servings of water each day, more if you engage in light activity. In addition, caffeine should be strictly limited to 200 mg (about two cups of coffee) or less per day; if you do drink something caffeinated, make sure to drink two cups of water for each cup of caffeinated beverage. Your diet should include plenty of fresh fruit and vegetables, with adequate intake of the other food groups, in order to provide the right supply of vitamins and minerals as well as fiber and energy to your system.

Apart from these very important basics of adequate rest and nutrition, there are wonderful and simple ways to honor your body and celebrate the spiritual and physical changes. Self-care is important during all stages of life, but especially so when you are nurturing another life.

Try Cocoa Butter

Cocoa butter is a wonderful and sensual way of moisturizing and caring for your body as it grows and shifts. Magically, cocoa is associated with love and abundance. Cocoa butter is also widely touted as an excellent product that can help reduce the likelihood of stretch marks. This mainly derives from the act of keeping the skin of the abdomen well moisturized as it grows, but cocoa butter is an ideal product for this thanks to its rich emollients. (Drinking lots of water to hydrate the skin from the inside also helps.) Everyone's skin is different, though, and no single product will guarantee to keep you stretch mark free. Look for a lotion or cream with as high a percentage of cocoa butter as possible.

To use cocoa butter lotion or cream, pour a bit into your hand or scoop some out of the jar with your fingers. Allow it to warm up in your hand a bit first; there's nothing less relaxing than having a cool cream touch warm skin. You can also warm up the lotion or cream by immersing the container in a cup of warm water first. Massage it gently but firmly over your body.

Massage is a lovely, relaxing way to commune with your baby throughout your pregnancy, as well as to care for yourself and appreciate your physical state. Treat yourself to at least one professional massage during your pregnancy if you can afford it. Your body is working overtime to accomplish the changes, and your mind and spirit are also working overtime to keep up with those changes. Make sure your massage therapist has had training in massaging pregnant women, because the techniques and awareness are quite different.

Make Your Own Pregnancy Massage Oil

Why not make your own massage oil? You can buy the vitamin E capsules at the pharmacy. The jojoba oil and cocoa or shea butters can be found in natural food stores or online. Once blended you should store this oil at room temperature.

YOU WILL NEED

❖ 4 ounces jojoba oil
❖ Small pot
❖ 3 vitamin E capsules (measuring about 400 IU each)[*]
❖ $\frac{1}{2}$ ounce pure cocoa butter (or shea butter)
❖ Wooden spoon, chopstick, or Popsicle stick
❖ 9 drops lavender essential oil
❖ 6-ounce jar (or bottle) with cap

DIRECTIONS

1. Place the jojoba oil in the pot. Carefully slice open the vitamin E capsules over the pot and squeeze them into the jojoba oil. Place the pot on the stove.

2. Over low heat, carefully warm the mixture. When the oil is warm, add the cocoa butter (or shea butter). Stir with the spoon or stick until the mixture is melted.

3. Remove from heat and allow the oil blend to cool. When it has reached room temperature, add the lavender oil and swirl to mix.

4. Pour into the jar or bottle.

5. To use, pour a little bit in your hand and massage it slowly over your abdomen. Do not use excessive force, and do not use too much oil; a little goes a long way. Make sure you cover the entire abdomen area, reaching down around the sides as well. If you

are gaining a lot of weight, massage your buttocks and thighs and breasts as well. As you massage, visualize the calming energy enfolding both your baby and yourself. Do this once a day. To fully relax and for a wonderfully sensual treat, get your partner to massage the oil in for you. This allows your partner the opportunity to reach out and bond with the baby as well. Alternatively, you can add a few drops to a warm (not hot) bath.

This oil can also be used in the weeks after childbirth, as the body regains its shape and you lose weight again. It takes skin approximately twice as long to regain its shape as it takes the muscle and flesh underneath, so continue to care for the skin of your abdomen. Do not massage your breasts with this oil if you are breastfeeding, as the baby will end up ingesting it.

*NOTE: Vitamin E oil is often applied as a treatment for the prevention of stretch marks during pregnancy. However, according to a study published in the *British Journal of General Practice* in 2013, there is no confirmed evidence that topical oils prevent stretch marks. In addition, vitamin E oil may cause a mild to moderate allergic skin reaction known as contact dermatitis. It may cause the skin to appear inflamed, dry, or flaky, and to become intensely itchy. Consult your doctor if you have concerns about the safety of applying vitamin E during your pregnancy.

Maternity Clothes

It's one of the facts of pregnancy that your body begins to change shape even before your scale begins to show a weight gain. Things don't fit quite the way they once did. At the same time, however, your body won't have changed enough to merit buying maternity clothes, which are designed for women approximately one-third to halfway through their pregnancy. (If you're on your second or later pregnancy, you may need to start wearing maternity clothes earlier, because your body already knows where it has to go and jumps ahead.) Don't be too eager to start wearing maternity clothes; you'll get remarkably tired of them by the time your due date rolls around! If you buy them too early, they may not fit you later when you really need them. Maternity clothes tend to be expensive, which is frustrating when you think about how little time you end up wearing them in the grand scheme of life. Most moms are happy to lend out their maternity wardrobes, so ask family and friends if they have anything in your size.

What we wear is usually very important to our mood. We choose specific colors, styles, and cuts to reflect how we feel, or how we want to feel. It's no different during pregnancy. We're fortunate that today's maternity fashions have moved past the jumper and smock fixation. These days, you'll find everything from jeans to halter tops, from dinner suits to cocktail dresses, and the cut doesn't try to hide the pregnancy: On the contrary, it celebrates your pregnancy. Stretchy fabrics and clinging cuts now reveal your changing body.

Make a point of at least trying on some of the clingier, curvy pregnancy fashions you find. Look at yourself in the fitting room mirror and appreciate what you see. Even if you aren't comfortable purchasing them or wearing them in public, the experience of seeing yourself clothed this way can boost your morale. Take pride in the curves, in the swelling abdomen and breasts, in the changing shape: These are what physically define you as a life-bearing vessel, as a living avatar of the Goddess in her guise of the Great Mother.

Aromatherapy to Cope with Changes

Aromatherapy is the practice of using natural oils to influence the emotional state. It functions by affecting the physical body via its interaction with the chemical substances of the oils. The easiest way to use aromatherapy to affect your mood is to put a drop or two on a cotton ball and carry it in a sealable sandwich bag to inhale when you feel the need for a lift.

Many people already use oil warmers, a dish suspended over a candle, in which a bit of water and a drop or two of essential oil are placed. This releases the oil's scent and chemicals into the air of the room. Scented candles are another easy way to employ aromatherapy.

Like any other physiology-affecting substance, essential oils carry some danger when used during pregnancy or while breastfeeding. Here's a list of what's safe to use, whether to inhale or on the body. As always, using them on the body means you're absorbing them into your body, and essential oils can irritate or damage skin if used undiluted. Always dilute essential oils in a carrier oil such as jojoba, grapeseed, or sweet almond oil before applying them to the skin. A safe dilution is usually approximately six to ten drops essential oil to 1 ounce of carrier oil. If you have sensitive skin, or an established sensitivity to any of these oils, don't use them at all.

Safe Essential Oils to Use for Aromatherapy During Pregnancy

❖ Bergamot (*Citrus bergamia*)
❖ Eucalyptus (*Eucalyptus globulus*)
❖ Frankincense (*Boswellia carterii*)
❖ Lavender (*Lavendula augustifolia*)
❖ Lemon (*Citrus limon*)

- ❖ Mandarin (*Citrus reticulata*)
- ❖ Neroli (*Citrus aurantium*)
- ❖ Peppermint (*Mentha piperita*)
- ❖ Petitgrain (*Citrus aurantium* var. *amara*)
- ❖ Rose (*Rosa damascena*—usually found in a diluted form of approximately 7 percent)
- ❖ Sandalwood (*Santalum album*)
- ❖ Spikenard (*Nardostachys jatamansi*)
- ❖ Tea tree (*Melaleuca alternifolia*)
- ❖ Ylang-ylang (*Cananga odorata*)

Ritual for Safe Pregnancy

Throughout your pregnancy, you are sent for tests, see doctors and other health professionals, and are made aware of the things that may go wrong. That awareness can sometimes get you down, adding to your already over-full plate of stress and worry as you balance your work, your family, and the needs of your body and spirit throughout the pregnancy.

Additionally, if you are very sensitive to energy, you may be concerned that foreign energies may influence or harm your child. In addition to shielding regularly (see Chapter 5), a spell such as this one can serve to defend the child from unwanted energy. Performing a ritual or spell to safeguard your pregnancy can be just the thing to help reassure you by adding an extra level of protection. This ritual calls on both the God and the Goddess as guardians.

The egg in this ritual must not be hard-boiled. The idea is to use the egg as a focus for the pregnancy, to represent the fragility of the life that is forming. To hard-boil the egg is to symbolically remove the potential for life. If you do not have lavender and/or sandalwood oil, use plain olive oil to anoint the egg. Sandalwood is indicated for its associations with protection, serenity, and success, while lavender is indicated for its associations of protection, peace, children, and stress relief. Olive oil is generally recognized as being sacred and can be used as a substitute for any anointing oil.

YOU WILL NEED

- Green candle in candleholder
- Red candle in candleholder
- Matches or a lighter
- An egg (do not hard-boil)
- Sandalwood oil
- Lavender oil
- A flowerpot (terra-cotta)
- Rich potting soil

DIRECTIONS

1. Create sacred space as per your customary practice.

2. Invoke the God as you light the green candle:
   Strong Lord of Day,
   Be here as I wrap a mantle of protection around myself
   and my baby
   To safeguard this pregnancy.
   I invite you to be present,
   And to lend your protection to us.
   I welcome you to this sacred space.

3. Invoke the Goddess as you light the red candle:
   Strong Queen of Night,
   Be here as I wrap a mantle of protection around myself
   and my baby
   To safeguard this pregnancy.
   I invite you to be present,

> *And to shelter us.*
> *I welcome you to this sacred space.*

4. Hold the egg with the small end up. Take a drop of sandalwood oil on your finger and touch it to the top of the egg, then the bottom. Dip your finger in the lavender oil and draw the rune Algiz on one side of the egg. Algiz is a protective rune, and also encompasses the concept of growth in safety.

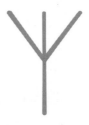

5. Fill the pot halfway with potting soil. Hold your hands over it and close your eyes. Visualize a white light beaming from your hands and bathing the soil and pot with its luminescence. Visualize any negative energy or energy not supportive of your goal departing.

6. Pick up the egg and touch it gently to your abdomen, then to your heart. Gently place the egg in the center of the pot. Cover it with more potting soil. Say:

> *Sacred egg,*
> *Symbol of life,*
> *You who hold a universe of potential within your shell,*
> *Be protected by this earth,*
> *This stable earth, which offers you shelter and security.*
> *Rest here in safety.*
> *May my child likewise rest safely.*
> *So mote it be.*

7. On the surface of the soil, draw the Algiz rune again with your finger. As you do so, visualize protective energy pouring from your finger into the earth, surrounding the egg.

8. Place the pot in a safe place. Once a week (a Sunday, Monday, or Tuesday are ideal) place your hands over it and strengthen

the protection you have wrapped around it. Be very, very careful to not knock the pot over; if the egg breaks not only is the spell likewise broken, which means you'll have to start all over again, but it will smell rather unpleasant! If the egg (and thus the spell) does break during your pregnancy, don't worry; just redo the spell with a new egg.

9. Once you've had your baby, take the soil and the egg and bury it somewhere with thanks. Be gentle as you pull the earth out of the pot and place it and the egg in the ground; don't break the egg. Pour a small libation of milk over the place of burial as a thank-you.

Chapter 7

Dealing with Unexpected Events

Pregnancy, being a natural thing, is rarely perfect. We are fortunate to live in a time when medical care can perceive a problem during pregnancy before it grows out of hand. No matter how advanced medicine and support techniques are, however, there are times when your pregnancy doesn't go the way you expect it to go. This chapter will discuss how you can deal with unexpected pregnancy concerns and the changes that they bring.

Bed Rest

Being ordered to stay in bed can be a severe blow to your plans. Whatever your circumstances—you may already be caring for a toddler or working full-time—it won't be easy to spend one or more months sitting or lying down simply waiting for your baby to be born.

Orders for bed rest can come about as a result of a number of things such as cervical issues, blood pressure, or preterm labor. Bed rest can range from being allowed to be up for part of the day doing light activity but spending a specified number of hours sitting or lying down (sometimes known as partial bed rest); full-time bed rest at home; and being in a hospital bed. Bed rest reduces the pressure of the baby on the cervix, which can reduce the risk of preterm labor, and increases blood flow in the placenta, providing the baby with as much oxygen as possible. Bed rest can be for a limited period of time, or until you deliver your baby.

Bed rest can be incredibly emotionally and spiritually challenging. Most of the time you feel healthy and perfectly well, and chafe at the thought of spending all your time confined to your sofa or in your bedroom. It doesn't help that your work colleagues or management may not understand what's happening, or accuse you of trying to take a free vacation, making you feel guilty for failing them in some way.

It is important to understand that bed rest is not a sign of failure or weakness in any way, shape, or form. While you can know this intellectually, it can be very difficult to understand it emotionally. Prayer and meditation can offer you the opportunity to explore your feelings regarding the situation. In the meantime, use your spiritual pregnancy journal to pour out thoughts and emotional responses.

You will need to ask for help. This can be the most challenging aspect of bed rest: feeling completely healthy but having to ask someone else to come in to watch your children, clean the house, and so forth. It can be difficult to release this kind of responsibility to someone else, let alone admit that you need the support. Friends and family are usually glad to help. Make sure to do something nice for them as a thank-you; often, a card or small gift such as candles or a bottle of wine is more than enough. Some women can continue to work from home, calling in or connecting to their workplace via the Internet. If your job does not allow for this, explore your healthcare benefits and insurance options for medical conditions.

Give yourself a break regarding your relationship with your partner as well. Tempers can flare and resentment can build on both sides in a situation like this. Be open and communicative about your feelings about the circumstances, and be accepting of your partner's emotions as well.

In the end, this is all for the health and benefit of your baby. Use the time to commune with him or her. Use or borrow a laptop and write letters, or a novel! Organize scrapbooks, sort through photos, draw and paint, work on crafts, or read. Create a spiritually nurturing environment around where you're resting with pictures and colors that relax and soothe you. Move your pregnancy shrine into that environment. Use a lap desk or a breakfast tray as a work surface and moveable altar. If you want to work with elemental representations at this altar and are worried about water slopping or the fire hazard of candles and incense in bed, use small cards with elemental symbols drawn on them (see the Appendix). Keep as many necessities nearby as you can to minimize the amount of moving around you'll have to do. Check with your medical professional for light exercises and stretches you can do in bed, and change position frequently to keep blood circulating and muscles as toned as possible.

If you are ordered to bed rest in the hospital, you'll be even more challenged to maintain a positive outlook. For most of us, a hospital means sick people, and the emotional and spiritual resonance of a place like that can be quite depressing. It's one thing to be on bed rest in your own home, but to be confined to bed in a strange place away from the home environment that makes you feel safe and comfortable, with none of your personal items, can be disheartening. In a case like this, it's even more important to keep yourself emotionally and spiritually positive to combat the feelings of isolation and alienation.

Again, call on your support team to help make the experience tolerable. Invite friends in to sit with you every day. Play board games with them. Read. Send someone to your house with a list of items you want and/or need with you, and make sure your telephone and address book are on that list. Don't feel shy about asking for fruit or treats, or for library materials. If you try to be a martyr or to be heroic, you'll end up lonely and depressed. Staying in touch with the rest of the world will help your outlook. And if you want time alone now and then, that's all right too.

Preterm Labor and Delivery

Sometimes pregnancy is unexpectedly cut short by your own body. Labor can be triggered by a variety of different things, or in some cases must be induced in order to safeguard the health of mother or baby.

When you are expecting your spiritual journey to last approximately nine months as most pregnancies do, to have some of it stolen from you can be disconcerting to say the least. In addition, those final weeks wherein you were planning to handle certain issues are suddenly rescheduled with caring for a preterm baby, either at home or in the hospital. This sudden acceleration of your schedule will of course cause an equivalent increase in stress, as you are thrust into a new situation without having had the proper time to prepare yourself spiritually or emotionally.

No matter what your circumstances, remember to take the time by yourself to think about your situation and to recognize your feelings about it all. Meditate; talk to the mother goddess with whom you are working throughout your pregnancy; appeal to the deities with whom you work for support, love, and aid. Journal your emotions, and don't feel guilty or upset if they're a convoluted and contradictory mess: Emotions by their very nature are not logical, but they are still valid, no matter what they are.

Infant Hospitalization

The first few weeks after birthing can be insane enough, but if your baby is still in the hospital you can be completely torn between home and heart. The hospital environment can be intimidating, and so unlike the warm cozy home you have dreamed of presenting to your child. You may feel a powerful need to hold your child, nurse it, and protect it. This may be impossible if the medical situation calls for the child to be in an incubator, or in isolation.

It can be completely counter to instinct to walk away from your child's bedside, to leave the hospital, but it's in your best interest to do so. The hospital staff is fully trained to soothe and care tenderly for infants in these situations, and your presence, while appreciated, can sometimes impede them from administering the care required. You need to reconnect with the world and remove yourself from the hospital environment to provide your spirit with a different context for a period of time. If you leave for a time, it doesn't mean that you don't care. That may sound obvious, but when you're in the situation, obvious takes a back seat to the driving need to be with your newly born child. Go out for a walk; go out for a meal with your partner; go see a movie. If you forget your child for a moment or two or even longer, you're not a bad mother. It allows your mind and spirit to take a break, so you can take a much-needed step away from the situation to reset yourself to a level more capable of handling the demands of the situation.

If for some reason your child must be transferred to a hospital in another city to receive the level of care he or she requires, you will have to deal with another spiritual and emotional challenge. For a variety of reasons it isn't always possible for you to travel to be with your child full-time. When this happens, set aside time every day to create sacred space and do a ritual to raise and send your child loving energy, or simply to meditate and commune with your baby the way you did while you were pregnant. As your child is literally flesh of your flesh, and has spent months gestating in your own body, there exists a link between you that can never be severed. You no longer need to be in physical contact with him or her in order to communicate; you merely have to reach out with the intent of contacting him or her, and your love and energy will connect. If you wish to leave something physical with the baby that has been empowered with energy for healing and comfort, you can empower a soft stuffed toy to send with him or her. Ask if the neonatal unit will allow you to leave photographs on or near the incubator or crib so that your baby will have a visual reminder of you as well, and ask what the rules may be regarding bedding and toys in general. All these things can be empowered, or serve as a focus for you through which to also contact the child. The opportunities you will have to travel and spend time with your baby, be it weekly or some other schedule, will still be sweet and special, and very valuable for all of you. With the spiritual bond you have formed throughout your pregnancy, you have a special connection to your child that allows you to be with him or her in spirit whenever you feel the need to do so, even if you cannot be there physically.

Even if your child stays in your local hospital, staying with her or him every minute of the day isn't healthy for you, spiritually or otherwise. You need to recharge, to change your perspective. Go home and work on the baby's room. Catch up on all the things that you need to have tied up before the baby comes home. Remember to ground and rebalance your personal energy frequently, or you may drain yourself unintentionally. As difficult as it may be for you, try to sleep as much as possible as well.

You may be dealing with feelings of guilt, likely unfounded, wondering what you did to precipitate premature labor, or how you failed as a mother carrying a child to term. To help you deal with the multiple levels of guilt involved with having an infant in the hospital (Is there something I could have done differently? How could I simply leave him/her there? Am I a bad mother already?), meditate on the following concepts. What do these words suggest to you? How can you manifest them in your life?

- ❖ **BALANCE**
- ❖ **SERENITY**
- ❖ **FLOW**

While you meditate, use such aids as candles scented with sandalwood, light rose, or frankincense, or anoint a plain candle with a touch of one of these oils. As always, use caution if using essential oils, for they are absorbed by your body and can affect your lactation. Write down your thoughts and feelings in your spiritual journal.

Using Oils to Help Heal Your Spirit

Here is a list of oil recipes for you to blend and use in your journey through the unexpected challenges that can arise in pregnancy and test your spirit. You can anoint a candle with these blends, put a drop or two on a handkerchief to carry with you, or swirl a drop or two in a bath. Be careful when you use undiluted essential oils: They are concentrated plant essences, and even a drop can have a serious impact on your body. Once you have given birth, the danger isn't necessarily over: If used on the body, essential oils can impact lactation as well. Make sure to blend these in a carrier base oil such as grapeseed oil, almond oil, jojoba oil, or even light olive oil.

- ❖ **TO HELP RELEASE GUILT:** 1 part frankincense, 2 parts jasmine, 3 parts sandalwood, 1 part cedar
- ❖ **FOR PEACE:** 3 parts lavender, 1 part rose, 1 part sandalwood
- ❖ **TO SOOTHE STRESS:** 1 part chamomile (German or Roman), 1 part rose, 1 part frankincense
- ❖ **FOR STRENGTH:** 2 parts neroli, 1 part helichrysum, 1 part rosemary
- ❖ **FOR HARMONY:** 1 part lavender, 1 part geranium, 1 part cedar
- ❖ **TO LIFT SPIRITS:** 1 part bergamot, 1 part geranium, 1 part neroli

Creating a Baby Shrine

If your baby is in the hospital for some reason, create a small shrine at home at which to focus your work. This shrine will provide you with a point of focus for your emotions, and a physical place in which to allow yourself to release any pent-up emotion, stress, and pain.

A shelf in the baby's room is an ideal location for a shrine like this. Put photos of your baby, a special toy, books, and any ongoing baby-related spellwork (such as the sachet from Chapter 9) on the shrine. The top of the changing table is a good location while the baby is in the hospital, but must be cleared when the baby is brought home.

YOU WILL NEED

- ❖ A shelf (a wall shelf, or a shelf on a bookcase)
- ❖ Picture frame, with a photo of your baby
- ❖ Cards
- ❖ Flowers
- ❖ Special toys or baby clothes
- ❖ Blue lace agate
- ❖ Moonstone
- ❖ Rose quartz
- ❖ Candle (optional)

DIRECTIONS

1. Place the shelf where you want it. Clean it physically, then purify it through the method you feel most appropriate (smudging, a quick wipe with holy water, and so on).

2. Place the framed photo of your baby on the shelf, and arrange the selection of objects (but not the stones) on the shelf around it. Cards of congratulations, flowers you have received, and special baby toys or clothes all make wonderful objects that add to this shrine.

3. Place the stones on the shrine. The blue lace agate is used for soothing children, the moonstone is for the bond between mother and child, and the rose quartz is for affection and love. All three also have healing and spiritual qualities to them. If you feel drawn to placing a special candle on the shrine with the stones to add to the energy, do so.

4. Each morning when you get up, spend a moment or two at the shrine with your eyes closed. Send feelings of welcome, warmth, affection, and support to your baby. Do the same before you go to bed at night, and anytime during the day when you feel the need to (re)connect with him/her. Use the shrine as a place to leave offerings or the physical components of rituals and spells you have worked for the health and well-being of the baby too.

5. If the hospital allows you to bring home souvenirs such as the cord stump, or gauze that has staunched blood after a needle, bring that home and place it on the shrine as well. This helps provide a physical link to your baby.

Miscarriage and Other Pregnancy Losses

No matter when in a pregnancy it may take place, miscarriage is a tragic occurrence that wounds all the people involved deeply. It's thought that as many as 50 percent of all pregnancies end in miscarriage, most of them before a woman even knows that she is pregnant. Of pregnancies that do become successfully implanted and recognized, 10 to 15 percent go on to be terminated in miscarriage. If you conceive twins, one can be lost while the other fetus survives, leaving you with an even more complex set of emotions to deal with.

Emotions of guilt, grief, sorrow, and bewilderment abound when miscarriage takes place and can escalate to depression and desperation if not addressed or accepted as valid. If your miscarriage was due to something specific and environmental, or an external reason such as an accident, then you may also be experiencing feelings of helplessness and anger toward the cause. It is crucial to acknowledge and deal with these emotions as well as the grief, or you'll end up with a wall of negativity that will make your future pregnancies very difficult emotionally.

Some of the emotions you may feel are:

❖ **SHAME:** Did I do something to cause the death of my baby?

❖ **APPREHENSION:** Will I be able to conceive again?

❖ **FEAR:** Am I broken? What's wrong with me?

❖ **GUILT:** Why can't I carry a baby to term?

❖ **FRUSTRATION:** Everyone else can have a baby, so why can't I?

❖ **ANGER:** I did everything right and it still didn't work.

❖ **REMORSE:** My baby didn't have a chance to live.

❖ **RESENTMENT:** It's so-and-so's fault that I lost my baby.

❖ **GRIEF:** I killed my baby.

❖ **CONFUSION:** I didn't even know I was pregnant, and I miscarried?

❖ **SORROW:** I didn't even have the chance to appreciate the fact that I was pregnant.

❖ **RELIEF:** I'm not pregnant.

❖ **BEWILDERMENT:** What could I have done differently?

Every emotion you feel during the process of dealing with these events, both before and afterward, is valid. Don't try to shut them away or deny the emotions; you will diminish yourself spiritually, and can cause yourself emotional injury.

Grieving

It is impossible to assign a value to the amount a person has a right to grieve based on the point at which a pregnancy is terminated. No one can claim more right to grieve simply because she was further along in her pregnancy than someone else. In all cases, it is the loss of potential, the loss of the fulfillment of procreation, the loss of life. The later the miscarriage, the more time one has had to invest personal energy and effort into the pregnancy, and it is this that one grieves for in addition to the actual loss of the child.

Counseling is imperative. If you miscarry very early in the pregnancy, counseling may consist of talking with your healthcare professional about the experience, and a physical examination to ensure that your health is good. If you miscarry later on, a course of counseling sessions with a professional counselor may be recommended by your medical professional. Don't dismiss this idea because it's too painful to think about, or because you think you're all right. Yes, it's painful, but the counselor is trained to help you with the pain, and even if you think you're all right a counselor may help you uncover repressed or ignored feelings about the experience that you ought to recognize. Let the counselor be the one to make sure you're all right.

Taking the time to heal is also imperative. The emotional wound may be raw, but ignoring it isn't the way to let it heal. Care for that wound with tenderness and accepting. You will be emotionally fragile for an indeterminate period of time. As a result, the rest of your day-to-day life will be affected by your emotional state, whether you wish it to be or not. You may doubt your ability to conceive again, or for the fetus to develop normally once your pregnancy is confirmed.

Saying goodbye to the pregnancy, and the embryo or fetus or baby, or however you think of it, is important. If you dismiss it, or attempt to minimize your grief by downplaying the impact of the event, then you are doing yourself a disservice. The pregnancy has been a large part of your spiritual, emotional, and physical life, and to assume that everything will fall back to normal right away is unreasonable. You must take the time to explore your feelings, to assimilate the significance and consequences of the event, and to acknowledge the loss, be it unplanned or determined.

Ritual for Releasing a Pregnancy and Fetus

If your pregnancy is terminated, give yourself the opportunity to bid farewell to both the pregnancy and the child. Ritual allows us the means by which we can formally recognize our emotions and provides a safe and structured environment in which to explore our feelings.

This is a ritual of release. In essence, it is akin to a ritual of mourning as well, so be prepared for a flood of emotion as you work though it.

Allow yourself some time between your miscarriage and the performing of this ritual. Doing it too early will be extremely difficult for you, and may be too soon to allow you the full release. When you feel ready to let it go, or when you feel that the time has come to release it and move on, then do it.

This ritual involves the tying of a knot to represent the reality and existence of the pregnancy. Before you perform the ritual, get a good knot book from the library or look up instructions on the Internet and choose a knot that appeals to you. Practice tying it with rope or cord of similar weight and flexibility that you intend to use in the ritual to prepare yourself, otherwise you may find yourself frustrated in the ritual itself, which defeats the purpose. The type of knot you intend to tie will determine how much cord you need, and how many strands. You should have at least 12". Try to use a cord with a diameter of at least ¼", to give your knot some substance. If the cord is too thin, your knot will be too small.

YOU WILL NEED

- ❖ Representations of the four elements: a small dish of earth, a small dish or cup of water, a feather or incense (scent your choice), a candle and candleholder (a tealight or a votive is perfect)
- ❖ Matches or a lighter
- ❖ Small taper candle representing your pregnancy (color your choice) and a candleholder
- ❖ Lotus oil (synthetic is okay, and probably the only kind you'll find)
- ❖ Cord, preferably silk (deep red)
- ❖ Box of tissues (optional but recommended)
- ❖ Candle snuffer (optional; you can use your fingers)

DIRECTIONS

1. Center and ground. Create sacred space according to your usual practice. I suggest a formal circle for this ritual. If you are not accustomed to casting one, see Chapter 5. Light the incense and candle representing air and fire on your altar.

2. Call the elements to be present, beginning with earth (north):

> *Earth,*
> *Element of stability and support,*
> *I call on you now to be with me*
> *As I bid farewell to my pregnancy.*
> *Earth, I welcome you to my circle.*

3. Call the element of air (east) to be present:

> *Air,*
> *Element of knowledge and wisdom,*
> *I call on you now to be with me*
> *As I bid farewell to my pregnancy.*
> *Air, I welcome you to my circle.*

4. Call the element of fire (south) to be present:

> *Fire,*
> *Element of passion and life,*
> *I call on you now to be with me*
> *As I bid farewell to my pregnancy.*
> *Fire, I welcome you to my circle.*

5. Call the element of water (west) to be present:

> *Water,*
> *Element of change and flow,*
> *I call on you now to be with me*
> *As I bid farewell to my pregnancy.*
> *Water, I welcome you to my circle.*

6. Call upon the Goddess, and invite her to your circle:

> *Great Mother of us all,*
> *Your daughter calls upon you now.*
> *Join me here in this circle*
> *And be with me as I bid farewell to my pregnancy.*

Loving Goddess,
Welcome to my circle.

7. Take three deep breaths and release each slowly. Center and ground once again. Anoint the taper candle with the lotus oil. Light the candle and place it in the center of your altar.

8. Pick up the folded cord and pass it over the candle, saying:
With the light of this fire I purify this cord,
And consecrate it to this use.

9. Weave your chosen knot according to your directions. As you tie it, think about creating a physical representation of the memory of your pregnancy.

10. When the knot is complete, pass it through the smoke of the incense, pass it over the flame of the tealight or votive candle, touch it to the surface of the water, and touch it to the earth, saying:
By air, by fire, by water, and by earth I bless you.

11. Face north (earth), and hold the knot up, saying:
Element of earth, energies of the north,
I release to you my pregnancy.

12. Turn to face the east, south, and west, repeating the formula with the appropriate elemental association and cardinal direction.

13. In the center of your space, hold your knot up to the sky and say:
Goddess, I release to your loving heart and healing hands
my pregnancy.

14. At this point, speak from your heart to the Goddess regarding how you feel about losing your pregnancy. Share your emotions, what worries you, and your doubts and fears, and know that no matter what those emotions are, she accepts them and you:

She does not judge. Cry if you need to, or scream; whatever you need to do is fine.

15. When you feel that you have shared your emotions as fully and completely as you are able, center and ground. Hold the knot to your heart and say:

    I have released my pregnancy.
    It is no longer a physical part of me,
    But I will embrace the memory of it in love and tenderness
    Until the end of days.
    So may it be.

16. Extinguish the candle representing your pregnancy, either with the candle snuffer or by pinching it out with your fingers.

17. Place the knot on the altar.

18. Thank the Goddess, using these words or words from your heart:

    Mother Goddess,
    Thank you for being here with me this day
    As I bid farewell to my pregnancy.
    Your love and support are with me always.
    I thank you, blessed Goddess.

19. Release the elements:

    Water, fire, air, earth:
    I thank you for your presence here in this circle
    As I bid farewell to my pregnancy.
    I release you.
    Farewell.

20. Take down your circle or sacred space. Extinguish the candle representing fire on the altar. You may leave the incense representing air to burn until it goes out, or snuff it out, as you wish.

21. Place the knot on your pregnancy shrine.

As a coda to this ritual, you may now wish to dismantle your pregnancy shrine with respect and tenderness. If you choose to dismantle your pregnancy shrine, you can pack the associated objects away to be preserved as sacred to this pregnancy, or you may wish to dispose of them respectfully if they were connected to this particular pregnancy. You may find that when you next become pregnant you will feel drawn to using some of these objects again, and not others. Alternatively, if you wish to maintain your pregnancy shrine as an aid to further healing and new conception, leave it whole, or remove only certain items that you feel no longer have a place there. A memory box is a wonderful way to preserve the objects from your pregnancy shrine, whether for the rest of your life or as storage until you create your next pregnancy shrine.

Talk to your medical professional regarding how long you should wait before becoming pregnant again. Discuss ways to minimize the possibility of miscarriage occurring again, and implement as many of the suggestions as possible. Once you have confirmed that you are again pregnant, look at the meditation for a new pregnancy in Chapter 1, and the ritual for safeguarding a pregnancy in Chapter 6. Tailor these practices to your particular concern or physical situation, if you have a specific condition that makes your pregnancy risky.

Motherhood During and After the Unexpected

If you do not have a complete pregnancy, or if you lose the baby at any point, or if you cannot keep the child and gift another woman with the opportunity to be a mother through adoption, are you still a mother?

In spiritual terms, yes. You have partially fulfilled the transition that is the rite of passage from the aspect of Maiden to Mother. No one can ever deny you the truth of your experience as you have evolved through your pregnancy, because you have changed as a result. You have explored and experienced the spiritual and physical changes that pregnancy brings, and that has altered you forever.

By working with your pregnancy in a spiritual fashion from the beginning and crafting a relationship with the Mother aspect of the Goddess, you have been moving slowly through that rite of passage, which usually culminates in the delivery of a living child, ending the voyage in the new social state known as motherhood. Being denied that final completing act leaves you in an awkward sort of limbo: You have mentally and emotionally and spiritually moved almost fully into the role of mother. You can never completely return to the previous stage. Your work throughout your pregnancy has changed you forever. Society may not recognize you as a mother, but the Goddess and your own spirit know how deeply you have evolved and how much energy has gone into your evolution. You more fully know and understand the Mother aspect of the Goddess, and will forever be able to call upon her wisdom with more ease than before.

Grieving

While no funeral is a happy event, funerals for children are even more emotionally wrenching than most. The cycle of life is something that neo-pagans honor, but it is impossible to understand why a child is born to us and then dies a short time later.

Look to Ashleen O'Gaea's book *In the Service of Life: A Wiccan Perspective on Death* for its general insight into this important part of the life cycle, but especially in this instance for its chapter on children and death. While it addresses death and mourning from a specifically Wiccan perspective, there is little within the book that cannot be easily extrapolated to apply to a general neo-pagan spiritual path.

Like your emotions at other points in the cycle of pregnancy and birth, your feelings regarding the death of an infant will be contradictory, deeply felt, and impossible to predict, let alone rationalize. Above all, they will be valid, and they deserve to be acknowledged and allowed to run their course. And indeed, these emotions should not be rationalized, but felt in their fullness and depth. The life the child lived, whether it be only in utero or for a few hours or days in the world beyond, should be recognized and celebrated, for the child touches and changes everyone's life in some respect.

Placing Your Child for Adoption

If you carry your child to term and cannot care for or keep it, offering the baby for adoption provides the child the opportunity to share in the joy, comfort, and security that another family may be better able to offer.

If you make the decision to place your child for adoption, you will likely find yourself working through several of the emotional challenges outlined in this chapter. The Ritual for Releasing a Pregnancy and Fetus may be of particular use to you. Substitute the word *baby* for *pregnancy* throughout the ritual, and make any changes you feel drawn to make in order to personalize the ritual according to your circumstances.

Goddesses and Adoption

If you are placing your child for adoption and wish to work with a goddess throughout the process, you can call upon Luperca for support and blessings, on behalf of you and the child you are placing. Luperca is the wolf who nursed Romulus and Remus, the abandoned sons of Vestal Virgin Rhea Silvia, fathered by Mars. In Roman and Etruscan myth, Luperca is sometimes equated with Acca Larentia, whose husband Faustulus finds the infants on the mountainside and brings them home for Acca Larentia to care for them as a wet-nurse. In some myths, Luperca is a goddess of abundance. Sometimes she is called simply Lupa. The wolf is an animal of stamina, great intelligence, and awareness of community. Wolves are associated with the paths of teacher and guardian. For all these reasons, Luperca is an excellent goddess to call upon if you place your child for adoption. She can offer you strength, as well as reassurance that your child will be well protected and loved throughout his or her life.

Any of the mother goddesses in Chapter 3 can also offer you strength, support, and comfort in the decision to place your baby for adoption.

Chapter 8
The Rhythm of Labor and Birth

Labor and birthing are about rhythms. The process involves bringing several rhythms into harmony: your body's rhythm as it struggles to find a rhythm through which it can birth the child; the child's rhythm as it naturally falls into harmony with your body's rhythm to bring it forth; the rhythm of the universe as the age-old sequence of birthing a child is re-enacted; and the rhythms of the medical attendants as they care for you, allowing you to focus fully upon the energy working in and upon your body.

The Power of Birth

It's important to fully realize the multifaceted experience of birth and its power. You become both immensely powerful and extremely vulnerable when you engage in the act of childbirth. While pregnancy is a long, slow shift, labor and delivery encompass a transition that is unpredictable in its length, as well as its obstacles. You will feel simultaneously very exposed, and yet still a mystery. Even if you have never had a baby before, you will find yourself engaging in behavior guided by instinct. This is part of the wonder and the incredible spiritual side of birthing, a true spiritual mystery. Opening to and embracing that mystery and power can help you fully realize your current role as Goddess incarnate. Being in harmony with the feminine Divine at this point will help you feel more confident instead of being open to fear. That power in itself can be intimidating, but fighting or fearing it simply creates more tension that can interfere with the physical aspect of the birthing process. Allow the energy to flow through you, and allow it to help the birth.

Alternative Birthing Options

Neo-pagans are an open-minded group of people when it comes to employing alternative methods of healing and health maintenance, and when it comes to childbirth, their stance is the same. Depending on your geographic location and proximity to cities and populated areas, you may have access to a variety of prenatal care and childbirth services. These birthing options tend to offer the mother great freedom during her labor, allowing her to choose how to move, whether she wishes to eat or drink, her positions, and who is present.

Water birth is a method of delivering the child in a pool of warm water, attended by trained medical professionals. Proponents of the method claim that it is a safe mode of delivery and provides a less traumatic environment for both the laboring mother and the infant. It is thought that the warm water provides a degree of pain relief and relaxation for the mother, as well as a gentler transition for the newborn infant. The water of a birthing pool supports the mother's body, reducing the effects of gravity and easing her changes of position should she so desire. The warmth of the water also relaxes and softens the perineum, reducing the possibility of tears as the infant passes through the vaginal area. Some birthing pools are large enough to hold the expectant mother's partner and/or other birth attendant. Theoretically the infant does not risk aspirating water, as the first breath is triggered by removing the child from the wet environment, and for a short while the infant receives oxygen both from the umbilical cord and from breathing, which also clears the lungs of amniotic fluid. As water is one of the four sacred physical elements often honored in neo-pagan practice, this birthing option can be a very special one.

Birthing centers or clinics are places designed and furnished like homes or bed-and-breakfast inns. They employ medical professionals, but they are places where expectant mothers can feel more relaxed than they might in a hospital. The philosophy held by most birthing centers is of noninvasive techniques that aid the mother in labor and delivery, as opposed to following routine medical procedure as in hospitals. As birthing centers focus solely on catering to childbirth in such an environment, and work with only a very few women at any given time, they offer expectant mothers a more individual-focused care that hospitals cannot. They are a formal part of the healthcare system in most countries, and both doctors and midwives may practice there. As part of the healthcare system, they are associated with hospitals; thus, should a complication arise with a pregnancy, the expectant mother can be transferred to an affiliated hospital for the proper level of necessary care. Birthing centers also usually offer prenatal training and support both before and after the birth. However, like midwives, birthing centers only serve women with normal pregnancies and noncomplicated births.

Home births are precisely that: uncomplicated births that take place at home, usually attended by a medical professional. The main advantage to a home birth is that the expectant mother is more relaxed in a familiar environment, while the major drawback is that there is reduced access to emergency services should complications arise.

Birth Assistants

Neo-pagans are among those who are open to alternative medical professionals when it comes to birthing as well, such as midwives and doulas.

Midwives are re-emerging as a popular alternative to hospital obstetrical staff. A midwife is a medical professional who offers prenatal care, assists with the birth, and attends both mother and child for postnatal care. Midwives are trained to handle normal births (births with no complications) with noninvasive techniques that support the childbearing woman spiritually and emotionally, honoring her position and experience. A midwife is legally qualified to deliver a baby and can practice in any environment such as hospitals (in some locations), birthing centers, or private homes.

A midwife is by definition a medical professional. In order to become licensed to practice, a midwife must usually attend a certification program and pass an examination. In several countries midwives practice in tandem with obstetricians. Legislation, licensing, and other requirements may differ from region to region within a given country: For example, at the time of writing midwifery is still illegal under certain circumstances in sixteen US states.

A doula is a nonmedical birth attendant. A doula offers pre- and postnatal support to the mother, as well as being present at the birth, but is not medically qualified to deliver the baby. Doulas support the expectant mother throughout labor, providing emotional support and spiritual support if she is of a similar or sympathetic path. Research done on doula-assisted births as compared to births without doulas suggests that the support provided by the birth assistant can reduce labor time and the need for analgesics and medically invasive techniques. The support of an individual designated to attend specifically to the laboring woman's comfort on physical, emotional, and spiritual levels can make a marked difference in the birth experience.

Easing Labor

Walking, dancing, stretching gently, and swimming are all ways your birth attendant may suggest to help you work through labor. Despite the fact that contractions are muscles tensing in order to ease the baby down and out of the womb, excess tension in the body of the laboring woman can in fact impede the uterine contractions, creating an obstacle against which the contractions must fight. Here are two very simple methods of relaxing body and mind, which in turn can help you handle labor with more ease.

Massage

Massage is a method of relaxing the excess tension that builds throughout labor. It is extremely important that someone familiar with proper massage techniques perform the massage if you are looking for in-depth work to help labor along, because a well-meaning partner or friend may make things worse or cause a complication. In general, however, a light and gentle rub with massage oil should be fine if all you're looking for is emotional support.

The following is a list of essential oils that are safe to use during labor. You'll notice that included in this list are a few of the essential oils you've been warned against using during your pregnancy. This is because they are emmenagogues, or encourage uterine contractions, which you certainly want to avoid during your pregnancy but which are necessary to actually deliver the child. Remember that all essential oils should be diluted in a carrier oil such as jojoba or grapeseed. Mix and blend these oils as you desire, empower them for safe delivery, then make sure to label the bottle clearly and pack it with the items you intend to take with you for the birth.

Essential Oils Safe for Use During Labor

❖ Clary sage	❖ Lemon	❖ Palmarosa
❖ Geranium	❖ Mandarin	❖ Petitgrain
❖ Jasmine	❖ Marjoram	❖ Roman chamomile
❖ Lavender	❖ Neroli	❖ Sweet thyme

Massage techniques can be found in several holistic birthing books. Bring the book along to the hospital as well. Be sure to communicate during your massage, letting your masseur or masseuse know when and where you need massage and how light or firm a touch you want. Talk to her or him beforehand and discuss your projected needs and feelings. Although your assistant may be tempted to channel energy while massaging you, this is not recommended unless he or she is a professional. During the birthing process the introduction of foreign energy, no matter how well meant, can upset your own personal energy as it fluctuates and strives to maintain its balance. Instead, ask the assistant to keep any proffered energy available in case you should wish to actively draw upon it at some point later on when you are tired.

Centering and Grounding

You've practiced these techniques all through your pregnancy, and they will be very useful when you are in labor as well (see Grounding and Centering in Chapter 5 for a review). Just as grounding can help you with physical balance and stress, when done during labor it allows you to work with your body's contractions instead of against them. When a contraction commences, relax your physical muscles and allow the tension to drain into your connection to the earth. Additionally, making sure that you ground regularly during labor enables you to draw upon earth energy if you begin to tire and helps balance your mood if you begin to feel frustrated or afraid.

One of the benefits of grounding is that once you've made that link with the earth, you can literally feel yourself relaxing into that connection. It can help you feel more in control and less adrift as you work through the process of childbirth, as well as providing access to the power and mystery encoded within one of the physical symbols of the Goddess.

The Concept of Natural Childbirth

Natural childbirth is a phrase that encodes a view of childbirth as being undisturbed by modern medical intervention. It postulates that a labor and delivery unaffected by drugs, medical procedures, a cold and emotionally sterile environment such as a hospital, and so forth is a better labor and delivery, sustaining less physical and emotional damage to mother and infant.

I've encountered a variety of ideas regarding the spirituality of natural childbirth, and I'd like to make something very clear: Following a neo-pagan spiritual path does not automatically infer a need for natural childbirth, and natural childbirth is not automatically an indicator of neo-paganism. It is not necessary to suffer pain in order to be a "good" neo-pagan giving birth.

How a woman feels about the subject of labor and delivery is a very emotionally charged topic. There's a lot of judgment and prejudice about what's perceived as better. What it comes down to is simple: Your opinion is precisely that, your opinion. Just as someone else's opinion is their opinion, and it is valid for them, you, too, are fully entitled to feel as you do about the subject. Be as accepting as possible about the variety of opinions on the subject, have patience with those who tell you that there is only one true way to go through the experience, and be as informed as possible about the variety of methods of dealing with labor and delivery in order to make the best decision for yourself. (The key part of that sentence is *for yourself.* This does, however, also include your baby.)

The end result of pregnancy is a delivery of some kind. It hurts, plain and simple. How you deal with pain and physical discomfort (note that they're not the same thing) is unique to you. Some women will swear up and down that childbirth was nothing more than an ache and physical workout similar to menstrual cramps; others require serious analgesics in order to focus on the event itself instead of being overwhelmed by the pain they feel. Some may argue that the pain is an integral part of the experience, while others may argue that in order to participate in the experience the pain must be somewhat diminished for certain individuals. There is no right and wrong; the choice is fully yours.

Many prenatal classes and physiological techniques that teach you to deal with the pain of labor do so with the aim of distracting the mind from the experience of the body. Pain has become perceived as an obstacle to birthing, when in fact it is a perfectly natural element. Some people argue that pain distracts the woman giving birth, and if the pain is eliminated then she is free to focus on the actual act. However, with the elimination of pain (particularly by anesthetics and nerve blockers), some women admit to feeling more disconnected from the act of labor and delivery. Pain is a method through which our body communicates with us, and it is possible that much of the pain associated with labor is in fact discomfort and tension that our fears and uncertainties cast as pain. Whether you use analgesics or not, accept the reality of the pain, allow it to wash over you, acknowledge it, and continue. Don't fight it; it (or your perception of it) will only increase. In no way am I suggesting that labor and delivery are painless, nor am I attempting to dismiss the very real situations where some birthing circumstances produce more pain than others. After all, every woman's body is different and will react differently to the process of birthing, and every woman's pain threshold is unique as well.

There are no rules in neo-paganism that state whether medical intervention is a good thing or a bad thing. Certainly if you experience complications during your pregnancy, your midwife or doula will likely refer you to a hospital, and the techniques available today may save your life or the life of your child. The main concern with establishments such as hospitals and medical professionals who work there seems to be the lack of focused personal attention available due to the high numbers of patients who require care. Patients can feel as if they are being identified with their physical condition instead of as a thinking, feeling human being going through a stressful and emotional event. In a hospital setting, rules and regulations apply, and personal choice regarding how you wish your labor and delivery to occur can be limited. It is important to remember, however, that your childbirth experience is what you make of it. You are in control of how you perceive it and how you handle the spiritual aspect of it all. Additionally, through your spiritual connection with your child you have a great impact on how your baby experiences the process as well. If giving birth in a hospital isn't your first choice, know that no matter what the setting, the miracle of birth and the rite of passage it encodes for both you and your baby is still a life-changing and extraordinary event. Your experience is still perfectly valid and spiritual, no matter where it takes place.

Preparing Yourself for Caesarean Delivery

For many women, the ideal of childbirth is a vaginal delivery. This may be because they perceive this type of delivery as being more natural, beautiful, or the way "it's supposed to be done." Like other childbirth-related knowledge, it may be an instinctual preference. When informed that they must deliver by caesarean, then, many women are shocked and feel bereft of an experience that is rightfully theirs.

Caesareans are performed for a variety of reasons. The position of the baby may defy vaginal delivery, or there may be multiple fetuses; there may be complications or an emergency concerning the health of mother or child, necessitating the delivery of the baby ahead of nature's ideal schedule.

It is vital when a caesarean is planned that you go through a period of emotional and spiritual preparation. However, in cases of emergency, time is often of the essence, and a woman is not often given the time she would like to think through what a caesarean delivery means to her spiritually. Even in the short time available, however, it is important to reach a frame of mind where you can focus on the baby's comfort and welcome, preparing yourself to receive your child and offer it nurture and healing. In situations such as this, call upon the mother goddess with whom you have been working throughout your pregnancy, as well as any deity you honor and work with on a regular basis. Open yourself to the energy available to you and use it to cope with the challenge of the caesarean, and to soothe your child, who is being born via a method he or she may not spiritually expect. Speak with the obstetrical team and ask them to be as gentle as possible with the infant, for this is his or her introduction to the world.

As joyous as your child's birth is, you may also find yourself dealing with feelings of guilt or disappointment because of the unexpected mode of delivery. Acknowledge these feelings and accept them as valid. Talk to a counselor if one is available; don't be shy about asking the staff if there is someone accessible for this purpose. Hospital counselors are trained to support people in situations like this; take advantage of their presence to help prepare yourself. If your caesarean is planned, take the time to meditate and explore your feelings on the subject as you prepare, as well as to commune with your child.

Childbirth and Transformation

It may be said of pregnancy that it is like a shamanic journey, where the individual descends down to the underworld to be ritually destroyed and then reassembled as a new being, rising again to the land of the living after facing death itself, triumphant and with new knowledge that may be used to help others.

Not only the mother goes through this journey. The infant, too, leaves their place of comfort on a challenging journey that is physically and emotionally taxing. The act of childbirth affects the infant deeply, and they are far from being merely a "passenger." The baby participates in the process, lending their energy to it throughout labor and delivery.

At the very least, knowing that you have built up a spiritual connection throughout your pregnancy with your child gives you insight into the fact that she or he has personal energy that you have certainly felt, defined, and connected with as your pregnancy has progressed. This spiritual connection enables you to reassure and soothe your child during labor and delivery, consciously or otherwise. Together, you and your child complete your pregnancy with a delivery.

Not so very long ago babies were thought to feel less pain, be nearly blind, and not recognize their mothers; now medical research has proven that newborn infants see, hear, smell, identify their mothers, perceive and remember, think, act, and react with awareness. Infant intelligence and capability is astounding, and a thing to be honored and respected. The birth process has a great impact upon the infant, as it does upon the mother. The journey affects the child deeply and spiritually, a transformative experience that shapes her spiritually for the rest of her life. As you transition through the wondrous and primal rite of passage that is childbirth, know that you are not alone: Your child is with you every moment of the way, participating in the sacred mystery of the Goddess.

Creating a Spiritual Birth Plan

A birth plan is an outline for how you want your labor and delivery to be handled. The theory behind it is that during labor you'll be rather occupied and won't be in the right frame of mind to properly consider situations as they arise and make grounded decisions. In a very real sense, this is exactly what will occur, because your spirit and body will demand so very much of your focus, attention, and energy. The birth plan is your manual for dealing with various situations if and when they arise, prepared when you are in a safe environment and in a calm, supported mood prior to your labor.

The birth plan allows you to submerge yourself in the experience of giving birth without having to fight your body's and spirit's instincts to focus on a question the medical team may have for you. Preparing the birth plan is also a good way for you to think about every aspect of your delivery experience and to walk through it, in a sense preparing yourself for it. In so doing, you can also take note of the areas that you can explore spiritually, providing anchor points for yourself where you can refocus on the spiritual essence of the experience.

Ritual for Crafting a Spiritual Birth Plan

This is a very informal ritual. In fact, it's more of an exercise, done in the sacred space of your choice. Do this in your pregnancy journal, and don't forget to put a copy in your regular spiritual journal. If you like, make another copy and put it on your pregnancy shrine.

This ritual uses lotus incense partially for its associations with Kuan Yin, the goddess of compassion and of childbirth, and partially for its association with spiritual equilibrium, harmony, serenity, and insight into the soul. The candle is pale blue for its associations with tranquility, healing, and peace. Feel free to substitute another incense and candle color if you feel drawn to them.

YOU WILL NEED

- ❖ Pale blue candle
- ❖ Candleholder
- ❖ Lotus incense
- ❖ Censer

- ❖ Matches or a lighter
- ❖ Your pregnancy journal
- ❖ Pen or pencil
- ❖ Candle snuffer (optional)

DIRECTIONS

1. Create sacred space as per your usual practice.

2. Light the candle. Light the incense.

3. Sit down with your journal and think about what kind of experience you would like your labor and delivery to be, from a spiritual point of view.

4. Write down anything that comes into your head. Don't censor yourself or your thoughts; just allow them to rise, and write them down as they come.

5. If your mind goes blank, relax by engaging in the breathing meditation from Chapter 5. Some concepts you may wish to meditate on are harmony, peace, rhythms and cycles, nurturing (both for yourself and the baby), success, fulfillment, safety, joy, your chosen mother goddess, the concept of the Mother Goddess in general, the aspect of the Mother, and the quality of motherhood.

6. From the words and thoughts you have jotted down, construct full sentences affirming your desire. For example, if you noted down, "embracing fullness of life," expand it to, "I embrace the fullness of life through the act of laboring to push my child from inside my body into the bright world of experience." If you noted down, "touching the Divine Feminine," you might expand it to say, "I will remain in touch with the Divine Feminine throughout my labor and delivery, and afterward." The point of this is to give yourself positively phrased statements that you can focus on as spiritual points of reference throughout the experience, bringing you back to the spiritual aspect of the act when you become too distracted by the physical or by what is going on around you.

7. When you feel that you have created a series of positive spiritual affirmations regarding your labor and delivery, you may

extinguish the candle and incense or allow them to burn out, as
you wish. Dissolve your sacred space as per your usual practice.

Do not be concerned about memorizing this spiritual birth plan
you have created. It is in your journal in order for you to be able to
read it when you so desire during your labor. (Trust me, there will
probably be a lot of time for you to read and think.) Your spiritual
pregnancy journal will be a valuable tool for you to use during your
labor, to remind you of the spiritual aspects of pregnancy that you
have meditated about and worked with over the past months. It has,
in essence, absorbed all the energy of the spiritual work you have
done, and thus will also serve as a source of calm and support for you
throughout the process.

It's important to understand that there will be a point during labor
and delivery when you forget completely about maintaining a conscious connection with the spiritual aspects of pregnancy and childbirth. There's nothing wrong with that; it's perfectly natural, and is in
no way a failure. And in fact, even though you may not maintain a
conscious awareness of those spiritual aspects, the spiritual dimension
of what you are doing remains active. Your awareness does not define
it. Some may even argue that a release of the awareness of these spiritual aspects is essential, for the synthesis of the individual with the
Divine Feminine at that point creates what is sometimes referred to
as a sacred mystery, something spiritual that may only be experienced
and not learned or defined through other means. Your spirit will commune with the Goddess, just as your body enacts her original and
perpetual birthing.

Birthing Charms and Talismans

Making something physical to have on hand during your labor and delivery is an excellent way to remind yourself of what you want to be focusing on. Also, having these things physically present means that they lend their energies to the environment, enhancing your experience.

You may wish to bring some of the objects on your pregnancy shrine if they hold special significance for you. If you are giving birth in a hospital, at the very least you'll have a small bedside table that can hold your objects, but you may wish to be circumspect about what you bring along in the interest of privacy, or you may find yourself defending your spirituality at an awkward time. Placing them in a small box, perhaps decorated for this occasion, is a viable alternative. If you are giving birth in a birthing center, then you'll likely have more room and more privacy.

Worry Beads

Worry beads are employed according to the practitioner's needs, but in general they are used by laying the beads across the palm and gently rolling them back and forth with the thumb. An alternate method is to pass the string bead by bead from one hand to the other, counting each bead or reciting poetry or prayer, much in the way prayer beads of various cultures are used.

Waxed cord is recommended for this project instead of nylon filament or wire, for its thicker diameter and strength. The thinner the stringing material, the more chance it has of cutting into your skin if tightly gripped during a contraction.

You may select beads for their shape, size, or texture, or their material. You may wish to make an entire string of identical beads, or a string of varying shapes and sizes. If you decide to make your beads from stones, you may wish to select hematite for its grounding and protective properties, moonstone for its spiritual properties and associations with the Goddess, clear quartz for energy, or a combination of the stones listed in Chapter 4. Make sure the beads are not too irregularly shaped: Playing with the beads is supposed to be soothing, and the rougher they are the more they may distract you or catch on fingers and clothing.

Decide beforehand if you will string your beads on a straight string or in a loop. Choose also the size of the finished project: Will it be short, or a small loop like that of a bracelet? A long string, or a loop the size of a long necklace? This will determine how much cord you will require, and how many beads.

YOU WILL NEED

❖ Waxed cord
❖ Beads of a shape and color pleasing to you

DIRECTIONS

1. String the beads on the cord, visualizing serenity and calm as you do so.

2. When the beads are all strung in the pattern you desire, knot the cord firmly. You may form the string of beads into a circle, or knot each end and use them as a single strand. Beware: Your strength will astonish you during labor. Make the cord longer than the number of beads requires so that you can slide the beads loosely along the string. This gives the beads more freedom to move if

suddenly gripped in a hand during a contraction, reducing the possibility of the cord snapping and beads flying everywhere.

3. When you are done, empower the beads for emotional and spiritual support, according to your desire. You may leave them on your pregnancy shrine until you go into labor, or you may begin to carry them with you now to further attune them to your personal energy.

The beads can be carried or worn, or hung over a bedpost or the back of a chair next to your bed. Be aware that your medical professional may not want you to carry anything with you during delivery. Additionally, if you make the beads to wear over a wrist or around your neck, medical professionals may request that you take them off for your safety and the safety of others.

Birthing Pillow

This isn't a full-sized pillow; it's more of a small sachet to tuck under a regular pillow. Again, your medical professional may disallow bringing anything foreign into the birthing room, so this charm will work best on the before and after parts of actual delivery.

Make sure the fabric you choose is thick enough so that bits of herb don't work their way out. If there is a particular fabric you wish to use but it seems too thin, double it.

Each item in the pillow is there for a specific purpose. The bay is used to purify; the oak is used for strength; the rose petals are for love and healing; the raspberry leaves are for ease of childbirth; and the flaxseed is for protection. The obsidian is a stone associated with protection, strength, and truth, and sodalite is associated with wisdom, peace, and mental and emotional equilibrium.

YOU WILL NEED

- ❖ 1 small bowl
- ❖ 3 bay leaves
- ❖ 1 tablespoon shredded oak bark (or 3 dried oak leaves)
- ❖ 1 tablespoon dried rose petals
- ❖ 1 tablespoon dried raspberry leaves
- ❖ 3 tablespoons flaxseed
- ❖ Obsidian (not an arrowhead; look for a plain tumbled stone)
- ❖ Sodalite
- ❖ Rectangle of fabric measuring 8" x 4" (color and/or pattern your choice)
- ❖ Pins
- ❖ Needle and thread
- ❖ 1 strand of your hair

DIRECTIONS

1. In a bowl, blend the herbs and seeds with your fingertips. If you wish, you can tear up the bay leaves and oak leaves.

2. Fold the rectangle of fabric in half, right sides together. Pin two of the open sides together, and sew them shut with a small running stitch. Turn the resulting pocket right-side out.

3. Fill the pocket with the herbal mixture. Add the two stones. Wind the strand of your hair loosely around a finger and slip it into the herbal and stone mixture inside the pocket.

4. Turn the open edges of the pocket to the inside, and pin the seam shut. Sew the seam closed with a small running stitch or whipstitch.

5. Empower the birthing pillow by leaving it in moonlight for at least one night, preferably three.

6. If you like, you can decorate the pillow with fabric paint or ribbons. After the birth of your child you may wish to sew on a small tag with his or her name and the date and time of birth written or embroidered on it.

Lotus Charm

The lotus flower is associated with beauty, the sun, and the element of water. Its magical associations include love, protection, and opening of locks. These associations make it perfect to use as a birthing charm.

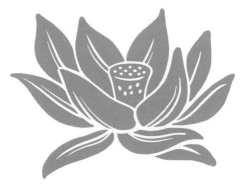

The charm is focused on an image of the lotus flower. You may use a pendant, a postcard, or a color photocopy of a depiction of a lotus from a book of Egyptian, Hindu, or Asian art. Or you may create a lotus image yourself, by drawing or sculpting one from clay.

The lotus is a symbol of rebirth and cycles as well, for it closes at night and reopens when the rays of the sun touch it.

YOU WILL NEED

❖ Representation of a lotus

DIRECTIONS

1. Take the representation of the lotus in your hands. Hold it up to the sunlight, saying:

   Sacred lotus,
   Flower of rebirth,
   Guide me through this cycle.
   When the time comes,
   Unlock the doors of my womb
   So that my child may be born in love and safety,
   Blessed lotus.

2. Set the representation on your pregnancy shrine.

3. Take the empowered lotus with you when you go into labor. Set it in a place where you can see it. At each contraction, invoke the lotus in your own words, either aloud or silently, and ask for its energy to aid you and your child.

4. After your child has been born, thank the spirit of the lotus for its help and support. Once you are up and about, you may either bury the lotus with thanks and a libation of water, or pack it away in the memory box in which you are storing your pregnancy shrine paraphernalia.

Your Newborn

Once your baby has actually been delivered, allow yourself the time to marvel at their perfection. You may be feeling tired and shaky, physically and emotionally exhausted from your experience, or you may be absolutely soaring. Whatever your mood, give yourself the gift of taking the time to explore the wonder of your new baby. After all, she or he is the ultimate gift from the Goddess, proof of your power to nourish and bring forth life. Marvel at the perfection of the tiny body, fingers, and toes. Admire and embrace the infant's instinct to nurse. Thank your gods and the universe for the wonder of this unique individual human being, a part of you for so long. Finally, at long last, you can see him or her, hold and stroke your baby with hands directly on their skin. And, gloriously, she or he can see and feel you as a separate being, as well as your partner. And above all else, give thanks for the miracle that you have participated in together, and know that the liminal stage of your mutual rite of passage is complete. From now on, you are mother and child, side by side.

Chapter 9

Postpartum Changes and Challenges

The period after childbirth, once you have brought your baby home, is an odd cross between bliss and despair. On one hand, here is the baby you have nurtured and communed with and anticipated for the better part of a year. On the other hand, you are tired and confused and terrified of making some sort of mistake. It is a twilight period, a liminal state yet again where you struggle to align the physical and emotional challenges of caring for a brand-new baby with the spiritual expectations of motherhood. It will likely be physically, emotionally, and spiritually exhausting for you. You do what you have to do, however, and a year from now you will look back and be amazed at how you met the challenges life presented to you.

Handling the Changes

If you thought that you went through a lot of changes while you were pregnant, hang on. Now you get to go through a whole different set of physical and emotional changes, plus deal with your expectations of what a mother is/ought to be. Handling reality as contrasted with your ideal of what a mother should be creates an incredible amount of tension. Look to the Goddess for a spiritual reality check. The Goddess has her moments of stress too. In no myth is she perfect: The goddesses of the ancients felt jealousy, anger, and resentment. When you feel these emotions, you, too, are the Goddess.

Life will change yet again. You'll wonder if you can handle being a mother, if you can live up to the role models you have consciously or unconsciously chosen, and if you have lost yourself and become simply Mother. The enormity of the responsibility of caring for this tiny and complex creature, who demands simply by existing, may threaten to drown you.

At a time like this it's good to sit down with your pregnancy journal again and look back at the list you made in Chapter 6 of what your definition of an ideal mother is. Then look at your list of what defines you as a person, as an individual. The former does not delete, erase, or replace the latter.

Rite of Giving Thanks

When the dust settles and the daze lifts you'll have a moment or two to look at the tiny, warm, scrunched-up bundle in your arms, and you'll be overwhelmed by a rush of emotion so strong you may wonder how you'll ever survive it. That emotion will be composed of many things, including awe, fear, love, and/or determination.

This is an easy ritual that you can do once you've brought your baby home. It is very simple and straightforward because once the baby is a part of your life, you really won't have much time for ritual. (See later on in this chapter for more on making time for your spiritual life.)

This ritual is designed to give you a defined opportunity to thank the Goddess for your experience of pregnancy, of labor and delivery, and of being a new mother.

YOU WILL NEED

- ❖ Birthday candle (in the color of your choice)
- ❖ Candleholder (a small lump of clay or dough will do, as holders for birthday candles tend to be designed to be stuck into cakes)
- ❖ Matches or a lighter

DIRECTIONS

1. Center and ground. Create sacred space as per your customary practice.

2. Breathe deeply and slowly to relax yourself. Take the time to reconnect with the core of yourself.

3. Light the candle and say:

Mother,
Thank you for your guidance, your love, and your wisdom.
I am (say your name here),
And I have triumphed.
I am woman.
I am the Divine Feminine.
I am daughter, and queen, and now I am Mother.
Your support and your strength helped bring me to this point.
Thank you for walking with me through this incredible
*   experience.*
Be with me as I move forward into this new life.
Help me remain calm and serene,
In harmony with my loved ones,
Patient and accepting of my humanity.
I offer you my deepest thanks for this miracle,
For the sacred opportunity to touch the very essence of life,
To cradle it in my womb,
And to labor to bring it forth into this world.
Blessed Goddess, enfold me in your arms,
And grant me your strength in the coming days and weeks.
So mote it be.

4. Sit, kneel, or stand and continue the breathing meditation for as long as you wish.

5. Dissolve sacred space as per your usual practice. Allow the candle to burn out on its own.

If you have constructed a pregnancy shrine, you may discover that it morphs into a baby or family shrine of its own accord as you place cards from well-wishers, photos, and new objects on it. This is a perfectly natural transition, and if you're comfortable with it, then there's no need to do anything else. If you wish to formally and symbolically mark the end of your pregnancy, you may dismantle the pregnancy shrine with reverence as part of your thanksgiving rite, or as a follow-up to it. If you wish, you may pack away the objects to keep them, or you may dispose of them with honor by burying them or releasing them into a moving body of water.

Additionally, make sure you take the time within the first three or four days after you give birth to write down as much as you can remember about the experience in your spiritual pregnancy journal. This will capture the incredible sensations and insights you felt during the process and chronicle your experience in order to round off the record of your journey through the experience of pregnancy. Giving birth is something that you will never forget, but the specifics of spiritual experiences have a tendency to fade from our conscious minds into our subconscious. By recording your thoughts and feelings as soon as possible after the birth, you will be giving yourself the gift of capturing your glimpse of that secret wisdom the rite of passage accesses.

Dealing with Postpartum Blues

Postpartum blues are not a joke or an exaggeration: You crash in the days and weeks after childbirth. Part of it has to do with the drastic and sudden shift in hormone and chemical levels that takes place as you change from being a living incubator to caring for something external. Another part of it is derived directly from the physical stress placed on your body and metabolism as your sleep patterns and eating habits go right out the window. And part of it comes from the mental and emotional stress caused by trying to keep up with the needs of a tiny infant whose main method of communication is crying and whose personal schedule is something unfathomable to others.

At this time, you may wonder if life will ever settle down, if things will ever right themselves, if you'll ever have a moment to yourself again. Your thinking will probably be fuzzy, and you'll doubt your ability to be a capable mother. Because you'll be short on time, and unable to take the time to do a rebalancing ritual or to sit and meditate—you're likely to fall asleep if you try, and that's not a bad thing right now—one of the best ways to help the postpartum exhaustion and tension is to use aromatherapy.

Aromatherapy is a wonderfully calm and direct method of influencing your body and mind. At this time, oils such as lavender and rose can help provide emotional balance for you. Jasmine can help you feel more comfortable with your body, and a citrus oil such as sweet orange or neroli can help you feel more positive.

One out of ten women experience severe postpartum depression as a result of these drastic shifts. If your symptoms include anxiety, sleeplessness, a change in eating habits, memory loss, feelings of grief and/ or guilt, loss of interest in regular activity and things that previously gave you pleasure, and withdrawal from the baby and your family, and extend for more than three weeks, please speak to your medical professional to ascertain if your postpartum blues are in fact postpartum depression. Depression can be treated, and the sooner it's diagnosed and treated the better for you, your baby, and your family.

Crafting a Baby Blessing Sachet

You want so much for your new baby! This little spell bag serves as an active energy magnet for all the good things you desire for your new little son or daughter.

The choice of color for this sachet fabric and ribbon is up to you. You can choose a color or pattern that complements your child's nursery space, or select a solid color for its magical associations. White is a good all-purpose color. If you wish to personalize this sachet, you can use fabric paint or embroidery floss to put your child's name on the fabric, or symbols of protection and success. If you choose to do this, do so before you sew the sachet itself: Fold the rectangle in half as directed in step 1 and sketch out where you want the symbols to go, then unfold the fabric and embroider or paint your desired markings. When dry or finished, proceed with the instructions that follow.

If you wish, you may do this craft in sacred space, or in a formal circle.

Make sure to hang this bag high up so that the baby can't reach it. Good places to hang it are over the window, over the door, or on the wall near the head of the crib.

YOU WILL NEED
* ❖ Rectangle of cloth measuring 8" x 4" (color your choice)
* ❖ Pins
* ❖ Thread (color to match fabric)
* ❖ Needle
* ❖ Iron (optional)
* ❖ 1 teaspoon dill
* ❖ 1 teaspoon birch (leaves or shredded bark)

- ❖ 1 teaspoon lavender
- ❖ 1 teaspoon rose
- ❖ 1 moonstone
- ❖ Narrow ribbon or cord, 8"–10" long (color your choice)

DIRECTIONS

1. Fold the rectangle of fabric in half so that you have a 4" x 4" square. Fold it so that the right side of the fabric (the patterned side, or finished side) is to the inside. Pin the two sides adjacent to the fold. Leave the third side (opposite the fold) unpinned.

2. Sew the two sides you have pinned, using a $1/4$" seam allowance. You will have a pocket of fabric.

3. Fold down a $1/4$" hem of the top rough edge of the fabric pocket, wrong side to wrong side. (If you wish to fold down the hem again to encase the rough edge completely, you may do so now.) Pin it down, making sure to keep it free of the other side of the pocket. Sew a straight running seam to make the hem.

4. Turn the pocket the right way out. You should have a square pouch measuring approximately $3^{1}/_{2}$" x $3^{1}/_{2}$". If you like, you can iron it before continuing. (If you have used fabric paint, read the paint directions concerning use of an iron before ironing.)

5. Place the dill in the pouch, saying:
   > *Dill, bring my baby good fortune.*

6. Place the birch in the pouch, saying:
   > *Birch, protect my baby.*

7. Place the lavender in the pouch, saying:
   > *Lavender, bring my baby restful sleep.*

8. Place the rose in the pouch, saying:
   > *Rose, bring my baby good health and love.*

9. Place the moonstone in the pouch, saying:

   Moonstone, guard my baby on his/her travels.

10. Gather the top of the pouch about 1" below the open edge. Tie the ribbon or cord around the gathers tightly, in a square knot. As you tie it, visualize all the energies you have invoked being sealed into the pouch. Wrap the ribbon or cord back around the neck of the pouch and tie it again, and then a third time.

11. Hold the pouch in your hands. Center and ground. Open yourself to the energy of the earth and allow it to flow up through your energy connection, down your arms, and into the pouch. Empower the pouch this way until you feel that it has been energized enough.

12. Hang up the pouch.

Making Time for Your Spiritual Practice

It's easy enough to say that neo-paganism is a way of life, celebrated simply by living. In reality, however, one of the hallmarks of neo-paganism is the performing of daily activity with awareness, understanding that every moment is in some way spiritual. When you're tired and impatient and feeling guilty because of those emotions and sensations, it's a challenge to open yourself up to the spirituality of the moment. The hardest lesson I had to learn once my son had been born was connected to my spiritual practice. I'd had a very rich spiritual life: I did ritual frequently both with others and on my own, researched and experimented, worked with two groups regularly, wrote my books, and taught classes on a variety of occult topics. When I was pregnant

I had to pare some of that away in order to conserve my energy for the pregnancy itself. When my son was born, everything was turned upside down. Because I rarely had more than fifteen minutes at a time to myself, I couldn't allow myself to get caught up in ritual as I used to; I couldn't go out to teach; I couldn't lose myself in research; I couldn't have a focused or uninterrupted coven meeting because the baby would wake up and need to be changed, fed, or interacted with in some way. I was left wondering if my spiritual practice, and possibly my spirituality, would survive my son.

It did, of course. Originally, my main expression of spirituality was characterized by a lot of service to others, communicating and challenging and facilitating other people's spiritual experiences, which is perfectly natural for someone who walks the path of a priestess and teacher. Having a child forced me to step back and look into my expectations regarding my own spiritual experience, and what I considered spiritually fulfilling on a very basic level. I had to streamline my spiritual practice, clarify what was essential, and classify the priorities in my spiritual life. It helped me sort out what I was doing because I felt it was my duty to the community, what I was doing because it was enjoyable, and what I was doing because it truly nourished something deep inside me.

The challenge isn't how to find time to fit your spiritual practice into your crammed schedule. Instead, it lies in thinking honestly about how you define your spirituality, your spiritual practice, and your expectations regarding a fulfilling spiritual life.

The following exercise will help you define and clarify spiritual practice as it relates to the unique circumstances of your life as a new mother.

In your spiritual pregnancy journal, write down the following:

❖ Three things that you feel are important elements of your spiritual path
❖ Three things that you consider indispensable to your personal spiritual practice
❖ Three things that make you feel spiritually fulfilled

It's okay to put the same thing in more than one list if it truly belongs there.

This may be easy for you, or very difficult. You may need to think about the exercise over a few days, or make longer lists and then narrow them down to three things each. The simple act of thinking these things through will be helpful in prioritizing what you consider important.

After a handful of days, go back and look at that list. Some of them may be difficult to do in the first few months. For example, if one of the things that makes you feel spiritually fulfilled is fasting for twenty-four hours while meditating, it's going to be impossible to do if you're nursing your infant. If you like to meditate and relax in a warm bath with essential oils and candles, then use this as a treat for yourself when the baby has gone down for the night, or when your partner takes the baby out for an afternoon. (As usual, make sure the oils you like to use aren't going to adversely affect lactation.)

In these first few months, even the time you take to relax and nurture yourself emotionally and spiritually can be tainted by the knowledge that the experience will soon be over and you'll be right back in the thick of things, as tired and impatient and teary as ever. The ability to focus on the present is a valuable tool in a situation like this. Being in the moment, and appreciating the spirituality of that moment, can enhance the spiritual nourishment that you gain from what you're doing to relax. Instead of thinking about how pointless it is to relax when you'll soon return to a state of tension and stress, embrace the moment and open yourself to the spirituality of it. Stay in the moment. Give it the respect it deserves by fully being there. If you think about what you have to do next, then you're not experiencing the moment fully with awareness. Take the feeling and that awareness away with you when your time of spiritual renewal is over. You'll thank yourself, and be more relaxed and capable of dealing with the day-to-day activity.

Nursing Challenges

The phrase *mother's milk* describes something simple and basic, perfectly suited for a particular individual, and the very source of nourishment and life. Breastfeeding a child is one of the many ways in which you can connect with the Goddess, for you are enacting one of her age-old responsibilities. There exist many statues and wall paintings of Isis breastfeeding Horus. With her strong connections to lactation, Brigid is another excellent goddess to call upon for spiritual support as you breastfeed your child.

While breastfeeding is a continuation of nourishing your child with your own body, as you similarly nourished your baby as she or he grew in your womb, it isn't as easy as it might seem. While both mother and child may have the desire to feed and be fed this way, much frustration can arise when it doesn't happen perfectly. There are several factors that can get in the way, the most basic being that both mother and child have to learn how to do it. Read up on it, talk to a lactation consultant in the hospital or local clinic, or contact your local chapter of La Leche League for help and support. If you'll be going back to work, look into pumps to express your milk to fill your baby's bottles.

Another issue that can arise with breastfeeding is a low milk supply. In theory, your baby gets exactly what he or she needs, but that isn't always the case, and most mothers worry about supply nonetheless. If your milk production is lagging, try taking supplements of milk thistle, fennel, blessed thistle, fenugreek, anise, verbena (also called vervain), or nettles, in the form of infusions or capsules. Make sure you're not sensitive to any of these herbs or oils, and watch your baby carefully to ensure that there are no ill effects on his or her end either. Dosages and recommended blends can be obtained from your lactation consultant or found in books or on reliable alternative medicine websites. Some women report successful increase or maintenance of lactation through eating a serving of oats in some form every day. There are various herbal tea blends on the market that can help stimulate milk production, or you can prepare your own from a recipe such as the following. Please remember: You should always check with your pediatrician before adding herbs and herbal supplements to your routine.

Nursing Tea

You need to drink an incredible amount of liquid in order to make milk on top of your usual hydration needs. Drinking this tea helps make up your required total liquid intake. If you prefer, you may use other combinations of the herbs previously listed or single-herb infusions to help stimulate your milk production.

YOU WILL NEED

- ❖ 1 teaspoon crushed fennel seeds
- ❖ 1 teaspoon vervain leaves
- ❖ 1 teaspoon nettle leaves
- ❖ 2 cups boiling water

DIRECTIONS

1. Pour the boiling water over the herbal blend, and allow it to steep for at least 15 minutes.

2. Strain and drink at the temperature you prefer. You may reheat it if you desire, or add honey to sweeten it.

3. Drink one to three cups daily.

Other Nursing Tips

To help stimulate lactation, aromatherapist Victoria Edwards suggests massaging the breasts with an oil composed of 2 ounces of almond oil, 6 drops of fennel essential oil, and 6 drops of geranium essential oil (do not massage the oil directly onto the nipple or areola, where the baby suckles). Additionally, meditating on images of fountains flowing with milk, or rivers of milk, or even of you nursing your baby can all help with lactation in general, and the milk ejection reflex in particular.

If nursing or pumping makes your nipples sore, apply a small amount of lanolin ointment to them to soothe the chapped skin. This does not harm the baby, and it really does moisturize the area and calm the redness. Only a tiny amount is necessary. Lanolin ointments can be found in the baby care section of your local pharmacy. If you develop mastitis or become engorged, try a warm compress of 2 to 3 drops each of lavender and geranium essential oils in a bowl of hot water. Soak a towel in this mixture, wring it out, and apply to the breasts.

If you must cease nursing or cannot nurse for some reason and wish to decrease your milk production, try including sage and basil in your diet in the form of teas or seasoning, or as warm compresses (follow instructions for the previous compress, using 4 drops each of sage and geranium essential oils). Again, watch your baby for any adverse reaction.

House Blessing and Welcoming Ceremony

As you have worked hard to be spiritually prepared for your pregnancy and the birth of your child, it only makes sense to spiritually prepare your living space for the new baby as well. It's also an excellent way to prepare your mind and spirit for the change in household energy, and to welcome the baby home.

To the Roman mind, the wild wood held the threat of darkness and savagery, and it was this influence that the deities Intercidona, Devarra, and Pilumnus were invoked to guard against. Intercidona protected the newborn from malignant spirits and influence, particularly from the malicious forest spirits identified with the wood god Silvanus. Intercidona, whose name means "she who intervenes," is associated with a knife or axe, or sometimes a large pair of scissors or shears with which she severs any evil attempting to attach itself to the mother and child. Devarra (sometimes Deuerra), a goddess associated with purification, used a broom to sweep the house of the new mother and child clean of evil and chaos. Intercidona and Devarra made a trio with a male deity known as Pilumnus, who used a pestle to bless the house and ensure that the child would never go hungry and would grow properly and with good health.

This house blessing uses the basis of this ancient Roman tradition to cleanse your home and welcome the new member of the family. As with many things that we plan to do before the baby is born, it likely won't happen until after the baby comes home, and that's why it has been included in this chapter. If you're determined to do it before you give birth, don't do it too far ahead of time or the benefit will be lost. If you are performing the ritual after giving birth, make sure there is someone else to watch the baby while you do it.

YOU WILL NEED

- ❖ 1 tablespoon dried lavender
- ❖ 1 tablespoon dried oak bark (or 1 dried oak leaf, crumbled)
- ❖ 1 tablespoon wheat berries (rice may be substituted)
- ❖ A mortar and pestle
- ❖ White or pale blue candle in candleholder
- ❖ Matches or a lighter
- ❖ A pair of scissors or a knife
- ❖ A broom (your besom, if you have one; otherwise, a new broom)
- ❖ A small square white netting fabric (tulle or organza would also work well)
- ❖ 12" narrow ribbon (color your choice)

DIRECTIONS

1. Begin by cleaning the house physically. Tidy up, sweep, vacuum, wipe down the counters and the doorjambs. Wash any dirty windows. Take it easy, because if you're still pregnant you don't want

to overexert yourself and damage yourself so close to labor, and if you have recently given birth you'll still be regaining your balance and strength. Ask your partner for help, or do what you can and let it symbolize a more complete cleaning.

2. Set out your supplies in the baby's room. Place the lavender, oak, and wheat berries in the mortar, but do not crush them with the pestle. Light the candle, saying:

    Let this sacred light purify and bless this home.

3. Pick up the scissors or knife and say:

    Intercidona, walk with me!
    Be with me as I cut away negativity and evil.

4. Walk counterclockwise through the house. Circle through each room counterclockwise. If you are using scissors, carry them open before you so that the blades meet and cut any negativity. If you carry a knife, hold the blade before you to cut loose any undesired energy. Walk with extreme caution and pay attention to where you place your feet as you walk with the blade. When you return to the baby's room, place down the knife or scissors with your supplies again.

5. Pick up the broom and say:

    Devarra, walk with me!
    Be with me as I sweep away ill-meaning energy.

6. Walk counterclockwise through the house once again, sweeping just above the floor. As you sweep, visualize any loose negative energy that is clinging to the area after being severed with the blade being swept away. When your counterclockwise circuit through the house is complete, return to the baby's room and lay down the broom.

7. Pick up the mortar in one hand and the pestle in the other, and say:

   > *Pilumnus, walk with me!*
   > *Be with me as I bless this house with abundance and health.*

8. This time, walk clockwise through the house, carrying the mortar with the herbs in front of you. Touch the lintel of every door with the pestle. When you have completed your circuit, return to the baby's room and lay down the pestle and mortar.

9. Lay out the square of fabric. Hold up the mortar again, saying:

   > *Lavender for blessings and peace;*
   > *Oak for strength and protection;*
   > *Wheat for health.*
   > *May all who live here be blessed with these things.*
   > *As I say, so may it be.*
   > *Blessings upon this house.*

10. Gather up the four corners of the square and tie the sachet closed with the ribbon. Hang the charm over your front door, or over the baby's door.

The Days to Follow

Now that you are a mother, in every sense of the word, there is a whole new world of spiritual exploration and discovery opening to you. As you learn and grow along with your infant, you will encounter challenges and obstacles that will test your spiritual strength as well as your emotional and physical limits. Indeed, the main spiritual challenge you may meet is that of finding time to maintain a spiritual practice in any kind of formal fashion. Focus instead on reconnecting with the spiritual aspect of everyday acts.

When your child is a year or so old, you may wish to begin taking a look at books on pagan parenting to explore ideas about how to raise your child in the context of your spirituality. Good resources include *Circle Round: Raising Children in Goddess Traditions* by Starhawk, Diane Baker, and Anne Hill; *WiccaCraft for Families* by Margie McArthur; and *Family Wicca* and *Raising Witches* by Ashleen O'Gaea.

Postscript

It is my deep hope that this book has somehow helped you throughout your pregnancy. Every neo-pagan path is different, just as every individual's needs vary, and thus the contents of this book cannot and will not be applicable to everyone. I urge you to use the information collected here as a basis for creating your own spiritual explorations throughout your pregnancy. I wish you a pregnancy filled with wonder, discovery, and joy.

❖ ❖ ❖

Appendix: Symbols

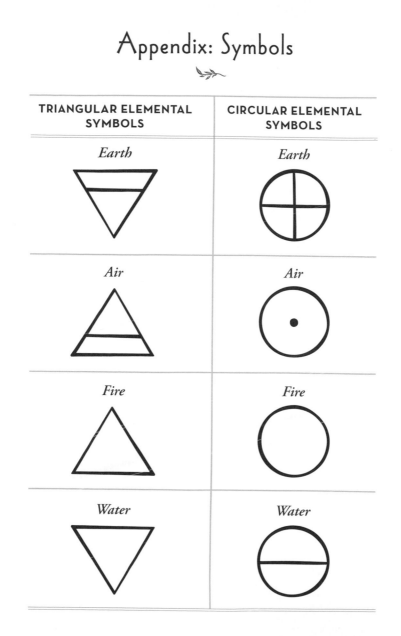

TRIANGULAR ELEMENTAL SYMBOLS	CIRCULAR ELEMENTAL SYMBOLS
Earth	*Earth*
Air	*Air*
Fire	*Fire*
Water	*Water*

Bibliography

"Acca Larentia." *Obscure Goddess Online Directory*. Accessed August 30, 2006. www.thaliatook.com/OGOD/ogod.html.

Andrews, Ted. *Animal-Speak: The Spiritual & Magical Powers of Creatures Great & Small*. St. Paul, MN: Llewellyn, 2002.

Beckwith, Martha. *Hawaiian Mythology*. (Originally published 1940.) *Internet Sacred Text Archive*. Accessed October 9, 2006. www.sacred-texts.com/pac/hm/index.htm.

"Eileithyia." *Theoi Project*. Accessed October 9, 2006. www.theoi.com/Ouranios /Eileithyia.html.

Ericksen, Marlene. "Aromatherapy and Child Bearing." AWorldofAromatherapy.com. Accessed September 19, 2006. www.aworldofaromatherapy.com/aromatherapy-article-child-bearing.htm.

Farrar, Janet, and Stewart Farrar. *The Witches' Goddess: The Feminine Principle of Divinity*. Blaine, WA: Phoenix Publishing, 1987.

———. *The Witches' God: Lord of the Dance*. Blaine, WA: Phoenix Publishing, 1989.

Forrest, M. Isidora. *Isis Magic: Cultivating a Relationship with the Goddess of 10,000 Names*. St. Paul, MN: Llewellyn, 2001.

"Gaia." *Theoi Project*. Accessed August 30, 2006. www.theoi.com/Protogenos /Gaia.html.

Goldsmith, Judith. *Childbirth Wisdom: From the World's Oldest Societies*. Eugene, OR: Closing the Circle Productions, 2019.

Harper, Douglas. "Virgin." *Online Etymology Dictionary*. Accessed August 26, 2006. www.etymonline.com/search?q=virgin.

Hobbs, Christopher. *Herbal Remedies for Dummies*. Foster City, CA: IDG Books, 1998.

Hoffman, David. *The Complete Illustrated Holistic Herbal: A Safe and Practical Guide to Making and Using Herbal Remedies*. Shaftesbury, UK: Element Books, 1999.

Holland, Eileen. *The Wicca Handbook*. York Beach, ME: Weiser Books, 2008.

———. *Holland's Grimoire of Magickal Correspondences: A Ritual Handbook*. Franklin Lakes, NJ: New Page Books, 2006.

Louden, Jennifer. *The Pregnant Woman's Comfort Book: A Self-Nurturing Guide to Your Emotional Well-Being During Pregnancy and Early Motherhood.* New York: HarperSanFrancisco, 1995.

Lust, John. *The Herb Book: The Most Complete Catalog of Herbs Ever Published.* Mineola, New York: Dover Publications, 2014.

McArthur, Margie. *WiccaCraft for Families: A Pagan Family Handbook.* Blaine, WA: Phoenix Publishing, 1994.

Monaghan, Patricia. *The New Book of Goddesses and Heroines.* 3rd ed. St. Paul, MN: Llewellyn, 1997.

Murphy-Hiscock, Arin. *Spellcrafting: Strengthen the Power of Your Craft by Creating and Casting Your Own Unique Spells.* Avon, MA: Adams Media, 2020.

———. *Wicca: A Modern Practitioner's Guide: Your Guide to Mastering the Craft.* Avon, MA: Adams Media, 2019.

———. *The Green Witch: Your Complete Guide to the Natural Magic of Herbs, Flowers, Essential Oils, and More.* Avon, MA: Adams Media, 2017.

"Nekhbet." *Encyclopedia Mythica.* Accessed August 9, 2006. www.pantheon.org /articles/n/nekhbet.html (site discontinued).

O'Gaea, Ashleen. *In the Service of Life: A Wiccan Perspective on Death.* New York: Citadel Press, 2003.

Roberts, Alison. *Hathor Rising: The Power of the Goddess in Ancient Egypt.* Rochester, VA: Inner Traditions, 1997.

Romm, Aviva Jill. *The Natural Pregnancy Book: Your Complete Guide to a Safe, Organic Pregnancy and Childbirth with Herbs, Nutrition, and Other Holistic Choices.* 3rd ed. New York: Ten Speed Press, 2014.

Starhawk. *The Spiral Dance: A Rebirth of the Ancient Religion of the Great Goddess.* New York: HarperOne, 1999.

Tedlock, Barbara. *Woman in the Shaman's Body: Reclaiming the Feminine in Religion and Medicine.* New York: Bantam Books, 2006.

Weed, Susun S. *Wise Woman Herbal for the Childbearing Year.* Woodstock, NY: Ash Tree Publishing, 1996.

Windling, Terri. "The Folklore of Rabbits & Hares." *Myth & Moor* (blog). Accessed January 24, 2020. www.terriwindling.com/blog/2014/12/the-folklore-of-rabbits-hares.html.

Index

INVOKE THE POWER OF THE DIVINE FEMININE.

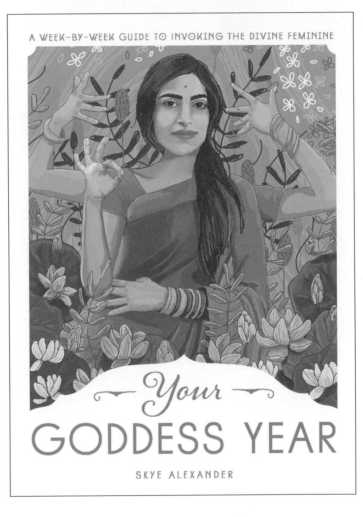

A WEEK-BY-WEEK GUIDE TO INVOKING THE DIVINE FEMININE

Your
GODDESS YEAR

SKYE ALEXANDER

Pick Up or Download Your Copy Today!

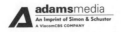